## Dedication

For my dad, with all my love.

# Contents

| | | |
|---|---|---|
| Acknowledgments | | vii |
| Preface | | ix |
| Chapter 1 | **What Is Raw?** | 1 |
| Chapter 2 | **Carbohydrates and Fiber** | 9 |
| Chapter 3 | **Fat** | 21 |
| Chapter 4 | **Protein** | 29 |
| Chapter 5 | **Minerals** | 71 |
| Chapter 6 | **Vitamins** | 87 |
| Chapter 7 | **Water and Hydration** | 105 |
| Chapter 8 | **The Effect of Heat on Nutrients and Enzymes** | 109 |
| Chapter 9 | **Understanding Calorie Density and Macronutrient Percentages** | 117 |
| Chapter 10 | **Nutrient Analyses of Various Raw Food Diets** | 129 |
| Chapter 11 | **The Importance of Focusing on Whole Plant Foods** | 147 |
| Chapter 12 | **Principles of Food Combining** | 165 |
| Chapter 13 | **Raw for Life: Helpful Raw-Food Success Strategies** | 173 |
| | **Conclusion** | 177 |
| Appendix • Helpful Conversion Factors | | 178 |
| Resources | | 179 |
| References | | 180 |
| Index | | 194 |

# Acknowledgments

SINCERE GRATITUDE TO THE FOLLOWING PEOPLE, all of whom made this book possible:

First and foremost, Bob Holzapfel and the Book Publishing Company for giving me the opportunity to make this book a reality. My editor, Cynthia Holzapfel, for your excellent suggestions and editing. Your vision for this book was invaluable in helping me hone my message to reach a broad audience. Beth Geisler and Jim Scattaregia for your respective proofreading and design work on this book.

Cherie Soria and Dan Ladermann for giving Dr. Rick and me the opportunity to bring our Science of Raw Food Nutrition curriculum to an international audience at the Living Light Culinary Institute on the scenic northern California coast. Our students, for encouraging me to write this book and for sharing the topics that mean the most to you.

And to my amazing husband Rick Dina, DC, thank you for your endless support and enthusiasm for this and all our projects. Your writing of the protein chapter, contributions to the fat chapter, and general editing were invaluable. We make a great team.

# Preface

THIS BOOK IS A HYBRID of the research-based information and my own personal and clinical experience that I've acquired since I became interested in raw, plant-based nutrition in 1990. I've included much of my own experience, because for all that's known about health and nutrition, there's still much that is yet to be known. On many occasions, I've had a question for which there was not a research-based answer, and it was my clinical experience or the clinical experience of other practitioners that helped me answer the question or fill in the gaps left by research. Clinical experience doesn't provide all the answers either, so I've found the combination of research and clinical and personal experience to be powerful for helping me achieve the health results I've sought and have helped others find.

Peer-reviewed research that focuses specifically on raw food is most certainly a work in progress. Given that there are so many topics in the health and nutrition literature that are not well studied, I encourage people to keep an open mind about their approach to health. There are many steps and tangents in between a raw, plant-based diet and the standard Western diet. Consider where you are personally on that continuum, what results you are experiencing, and how these relate to your personal health goals. Your approach to diet doesn't necessarily have to involve extremes or what someone else considers to be ideal, and just like research, can be a work in progress.

This book doesn't require that you have a previous working knowledge of nutrition. I start with the basics and build on this foundation as the book progresses. In order to clarify areas of confusion that people may experience, I touch on topics that are often misreported in the media or misunderstood. These include glycemic index and load, vitamins $B_{12}$ and D, and oxalates in leafy greens, to name a few. Throughout the book, I make distinctions among research-based information, clinically derived information, anecdotal or personal experience, and my own opinion. I think that it's important for people to know the source of my information and that I find information from all these sources to be very interesting and relevant.

Consider the following before you begin:

**1.** There is much useful information in this book, but it's just the beginning, representing a portion of what I've learned over the years. In a sense this book is a clearinghouse for the raw food nutrition topics I find most important for success, as well as those that are most misunderstood. Expanded information on these topics, as well as many additional relevant topics not covered here, are included in our series of Science of Raw Food Nutrition classes.

**2.** The information in this book is not medical, health, or dietary advice and should not be treated as such. The menu plans in this book are examples of foods and diet structures that I have observed in the raw community. Any type of dietary change or nutritional therapy should always be undertaken with the supervision of a qualified health care practitioner.

**3.** The nutrient content of foods in this book was compiled from the US Department of Agriculture (USDA) National Nutrient Database for Standard Reference and ESHA Food Processor, both of which provide the nutrient content of nonorganically grown foods, unless specified. I look forward to a time when the content of specific nutrients is measured in organic foods and reported in nutrition databases for comparison to nonorganic foods.

**4.** The foods analyzed for nutrient content are raw unless otherwise specified. To the best of my ability, I've omitted hard-to-find and expensive foods in order to give readers the most cost-effective choices possible. I would encourage those of you who live in areas where tropical foods are abundant and inexpensive to evaluate the nutrient content of these foods and suitability for inclusion in your diet.

**5.** The amounts of foods analyzed in this book are servings that are common for many raw-food enthusiasts. As will be discussed in this book, when someone starts replacing heavier cooked foods with raw fruits and vegetables, they generally eat a greater volume overall than they did previously, because fruits and vegetables have lower calorie density than heavier cooked foods (see page 120). If the serving sizes are too large for you, feel free to adjust them. If you divide a serving in half, simply divide the nutrient content in half to obtain the values for the new serving.

**6.** The nutrition field is not tightly regulated and is susceptible to trends and marketing influences that may lead to the dissemination of information backed by special interests. This can certainly be true with the sale of various health products. When I first started my health journey, I was amazed to see the pervasiveness of this type of information and how challenging it can be to sift through it in order to find valuable and accurate information. I've found my formal education in the basic sciences to be invaluable for gaining a better understanding of these topics. The more well educated you are, the more discerning you can be with the information you hear from various sources. It's my sincere desire that this book becomes a useful part of your education.

**7.** Nutrition is a field of science that's constantly under investigation by the research community and clinicians who utilize it in their practices. As a result, it's a constantly evolving field of inquiry. The information in this book reflects current knowledge of human physiology, biochemistry, and other sciences applied to raw food nutrition. Given the updated perspective of this information, some of what you read in this book may be different from what you may have read in other books about raw food diets.

**8.** Natural variation in the nutrient content of whole plant foods is common. I've seen differences ranging from minimal to significant among databases and samples tested. Because of this, I generally choose foods for individual and collective nutrient analyses that offer the best overall representation of nutrient content, rather than outliers.

**9.** When discussing the nutrient content of various foods, I've included various grains, pseudograins, and legumes for people who eat cooked foods. Some of these foods, such as lentils and quinoa, can be sprouted or cooked. Wild rice can be cooked or it can be prepared raw using a technique called blooming. Some are generally cooked, such as brown rice. If you have any question as to whether or not a food is generally cooked or eaten raw, I would encourage you to do some research as to how raw-food enthusiasts prepare them.

**10.** The cup and gram measurements for sprouted lentils in this book are based on my observations of green lentils soaked for 8 hours, then sprouted for two days (48 hours) at room temperature (68 degrees F). These measurements may differ from databases that report observations for longer or shorter sprouting times at higher or lower temperatures.

I wish you all the best on your health journey and encourage you to continue to learn and expand your knowledge base on this ever-evolving and fascinating topic of nutrition!

**Best of health,**
Karin Dina, DC

CHAPTER 1

# What Is Raw?

————— ∽∞∾ —————

WHEN I FIRST ADOPTED A RAW-FOOD LIFESTYLE back in 1990, I was thrilled by the health benefits I started to experience but was puzzled by the lack of awareness and information about this approach to eating and living. Why didn't more people know about raw diets? If these diets characterize a more natural way of living, then why haven't we been eating like this for millennia? Why wasn't this approach taught in nutrition classes at colleges and universities? Why wasn't there more reliable and substantial information available on raw food nutrition?

This lack of awareness astounded me so much that I felt I needed to tell people about my own healing experiences. It was then that I realized why raw food was not that popular. Most people were not really interested in hearing anecdotal information about one person's experience and were even less interested in changing their current eating patterns, because these habits seemed to suit them just fine. Not many people back then considered the connection between diet and health.

In the mid-twentieth century, processing and packaging of foods became very popular. The advent of these foods meant less time was needed in the kitchen, so people took advantage of this opportunity. These processed and packaged foods have become so much the norm that few people question their use. Anyone who avoids processed food as a way to improve their health is often seen as "different." A diet based on whole foods is now considered alternative. It's amazing how far we've come from what is truly natural.

Nowadays, there is much more awareness of the connection between food and health, and along with this awareness the raw-food lifestyle has become more popular. I'm very happy to see that people are looking for dietary approaches that help them reach their health goals. The popularity of various health care alternatives has also grown during this time. People are more willing to search beyond traditional medicine if they're not getting the results they're looking for.

There are certainly many answers to the question, why raw? Some are complex and some very simple. Although many of these answers are science-based, for Rick and myself, the simplest answer is that it works. A raw diet has improved our energy, focus, appearance, athletic performance and recovery time, sleep quality, and general sense of well-being. These experiences can be tough to quantify, but for us they've been notable. In fact, this dietary change has made such a difference that we decided to share our experiences and research with others through our series of Science of Raw Food Nutrition classes. Our goal is to give people an education about health from the perspective of the big picture and to also make sure they understand the individual elements important for its achievement.

Our raw-food journeys have certainly been varied, and admittedly we've tried many approaches to raw eating over the years, each with different and interesting results. So for us, understanding raw food diets has not only been about gathering information, but also about how to interpret it and put it together into a workable approach for eating in the real world.

This being said, eating raw is not the only consideration people make in their food choices, and we'll address this throughout the book. We see the benefits of a potential continuum rather than a diet that's either completely raw or completely cooked. While the focus of our diets is on whole plant foods in their uncooked state, we've found some circumstances in which cooking is appropriate, and this book addresses these circumstances. We also discuss the differences among various cooking methods, given that they don't all have the same effect on nutrients.

## The Definition of a Raw Diet

A healthy raw food diet is based on plant foods in their whole, natural form— food as it is grown. We think of eating raw foods as more of a lifestyle than a diet. The term "diet" is often used to mean an eating plan undertaken for a period of time with the intention of losing weight or dealing with a food intolerance or allergy. A raw food diet is much more than this, given that people embark on a raw-food program for many diverse reasons, including health improvement, a more youthful appearance, greater energy, environmental considerations, and animal welfare, to name a few. Just as there are many reasons for shifting to a raw-food lifestyle, there are as many approaches to raw food as there are people who eat this way.

If someone is eating a raw food diet, they're generally consuming the majority of or all their food as whole plant foods in an unheated state. These foods may include some combination of the following:

- fruits (sweet, starchy, or fatty)
- vegetables
- nuts and seeds (dry, soaked, or sprouted)
- grains (generally sprouted)
- legumes (generally sprouted)
- grasses
- sea vegetables
- raw condiments, such as sweeteners
- edible algae and cyanobacteria (such as nori and spirulina)

The contents of a raw diet will vary by person. The consumption of raw animal products has become popular in some circles in the past couple of years, but since our experience is with plant-based nutrition, we focus on plant foods in this book.

There are many different philosophies about which types of raw food are optimal, given someone's individual needs. Here are some of the most popular types we see:

**High-sweet fruit diet.** People opting for this approach obtain most of their calories from sweet fruits, such as bananas, berries, citrus, dates, figs, mangoes, melons, papayas, persimmons, and stone fruits. Low-sweet fruits (see the list that follows) are included, along with starchy vegetables, such as carrots, and nonstarchy vegetables, such as leafy greens and celery. Some people who eat this diet include varying amounts of nuts and seeds.

**Low-sweet fruit diet.** Someone with this diet avoids sweet fruits or keeps them to a minimum but may include other botanical fruits, such as bell peppers, cucumbers, lemons, limes, summer squash, tomatoes, and zucchini. This approach may include leafy greens, sprouted grains and pseudograins, sprouted legumes and seeds, avocados, nonstarchy vegetables, algae, grasses, nuts and seeds, and sea vegetables.

**Intermediate raw diet.** This diet is the combination of the high-sweet fruit and low-sweet fruit diets.

**80-percent raw (20-percent cooked) diet.** This intermediate raw diet may include some steamed vegetables and cooked yams, legumes, grains, and pseudograins.

## An Introduction to Macronutrients

In order to understand how raw diets can be nutritionally plentiful and promote health, you'll need a basic understanding of the nutrients in foods and how they work together. The nutrients we derive from food can be classified as carbohydrate, protein, fat, fiber, vitamins, minerals, and phytochemicals (such as antioxidants).

Carbohydrate, protein, and fat are considered to be macronutrients, since they're consumed in the greatest amounts and provide us with energy in the form of calories. They also serve as building blocks for the formation of cells and tissues throughout the body. Fiber, also considered a macronutrient, is the indigestible portion of plant matter that's often referred to as roughage. Although it doesn't make a direct nutritional contribution, fiber plays critically important roles in various aspects of intestinal health, blood sugar and cholesterol regulation, and weight management, in addition to other health benefits. The amount of a nutrient that's commonly accepted by scientists to meet the requirements for 97.5 percent of healthy people in each stage of life is called the Recommended Dietary Allowance (RDA).

Here are some helpful definitions:

**Calorie.** The amount of energy that we get from food is measured in kilocalories (kcal), more commonly referred to as calories. Your daily personal calorie need is dependent upon your weight, height, sex, genetic factors, and the amount of energy needed for movement and exercise. There is no RDA for calories, likely because of this variation in individual need.

**Protein.** Protein has both structural and functional roles in the body, where it is used in the production of enzymes, hormones, connective tissue, cartilage, bone, muscles, and organs, to name a few.

**Carbohydrate.** Carbohydrates provide energy for most cells in the body, are used to create the building blocks of the genetic code (DNA and RNA), can be stored in the form of glycogen, and have numerous other uses in the body. Nondigestible carbohydrate is also known as dietary fiber.

**Fat.** Fats contribute to energy storage, cell membrane structure and function, and cushioning of organs, among other functions.

**Dietary fiber.** The indigestible portion of plant foods is known as dietary fiber. An example is cellulose. Some functions of fiber include the following:

- keeping food moving though the intestines by helping to optimize intestinal transit time
- helping to slow down the digestion of carbohydrates, thereby decreasing their rate of absorption and helping to stabilize blood sugar levels
- binding to excess cholesterol in the digestive tract, keeping it from being absorbed and helping to maintain blood cholesterol levels at an appropriate level

## Macronutrients in Whole Plant Foods

All whole plant foods contain some combination of carbohydrate, protein, and fat. Even fruits contain both protein and fat, which is surprising to many people.

For comparison, red meat, poultry, and fish contain some combination of protein and fat. Dairy products contain combinations of carbohydrate, protein, and fat. The carbohydrate found in dairy products is lactose, the only sugar of animal origin. Measuring macronutrients as a percentage of calories allows us to compare the proportion of calories from carbohydrate, protein, and fat found in a particular food or group of foods. The water and fiber content of a food contributes to the food's weight but not the calories it contains. (For more information on this, please see pages 117–120.) Table 1.1 (page 6) shows the carbohydrate, protein, and fat content, as a percentage of calories, in a sampling of foods consumed by raw-food enthusiasts.

## Fruits

Botanically speaking, fruits are the portions of a plant that contains seeds. Fruits can be loosely categorized into sweet fruits and nonsweet fruits. Fruits found in the rose family, including stone fruits (peaches, cherries, apricots, plums, pears, apples, and so on) can be classified as sweet fruits due to their high content of simple carbohydrates. (For information about simple and complex carbohydrates, see pages 9–11.)

The cucumber or squash plant family has a number of fruits that contain more complex carbohydrates and are therefore less sweet. Examples include cucumbers, summer squash, and winter squash. This same plant family includes sweet fruits, such as melons. In culinary applications, nonsweet fruits of the cucumber family may be considered vegetables. Edible fruits in the nightshade family, such as tomatoes, eggplant, and bell peppers are botanically fruits, but may be considered vegetables for culinary purposes. White potatoes are also a member of the nightshade family and may be considered a root vegetable for culinary purposes.

## Vegetables

As a group, vegetables tend to be more varied in their appearance and nutrient composition than other groupings. Vegetables can be loosely grouped into starchy and nonstarchy vegetables. Starchy vegetables tend to contain more calories per gram than nonstarchy vegetables. For example, yams have more calories per unit of weight than leafy greens. Leafy green vegetables would be considered low in starch, while carrots are much higher in starch. Yams and white potatoes can be considered starchy root vegetables.

## Nuts, Seeds, and Oils

Nuts, seeds, and oils generally have the greatest fat content compared to other foods. Some exceptions include coconuts and avocados, which are grouped under fruits. There are several different types of fats in these foods, all of which have different roles in the body.

There are three oils listed in table 1.1: cacao butter, coconut oil, and olive oil. None of these three (or any other oils that have been separated from their whole food source) contain any protein or carbohydrates. In addition, unlike the whole food from which it originated, oil does not contain any water or fiber, making it especially concentrated.

**Table 1.1.** Macronutrient content of various foods

|  | Carbohydrate (%) | Protein (%) | Fat (%) |
|---|---|---|---|
| **Fruits** |  |  |  |
| Apple | 95 | 2 | 3 |
| Avocado | 12 | 5 | 83 |
| Banana | 93 | 4 | 3 |
| Blueberries | 91 | 5 | 4 |
| Coconut, mature | 16 | 3 | 81 |
| Dates, medjool | 97 | 2 | 1 |
| Durian | 67 | 4 | 29 |
| Lemon | 95 | 4 | 1 |
| Mango | 94 | 3 | 3 |
| Orange | 91 | 7 | 2 |
| Papaya | 91 | 6 | 3 |
| **Vegetables** |  |  |  |
| Bok choy | 53 | 36 | 11 |
| Broccoli | 65 | 27 | 8 |
| Carrot | 87 | 8 | 5 |
| Cucumber | 80 | 14 | 6 |
| Dandelion greens | 68 | 20 | 12 |
| Kale | 67 | 22 | 11 |
| Potato, white (baked or raw) | 89 | 10 | 1 |
| Romaine lettuce | 63 | 24 | 13 |
| Tomato | 75 | 17 | 8 |
| Yam | 92 | 7 | 1 |
| Zucchini | 68 | 24 | 8 |
| **Nuts, seeds, and oils** |  |  |  |
| Almonds | 14 | 14 | 72 |
| Brazil nuts | 7 | 8 | 85 |
| Cacao butter | 0 | 0 | 100 |
| Cashews | 21 | 12 | 67 |
| Chia seeds | 34 | 12 | 54 |
| Coconut oil, unrefined | 0 | 0 | 100 |
| Flaxseeds, golden | 20 | 13 | 67 |
| Macadamia nuts | 7 | 4 | 89 |
| Olive oil, extra virgin | 0 | 0 | 100 |
| Pumpkin seeds | 12 | 17 | 71 |
| Sesame seeds | 15 | 12 | 73 |
| Sunflower seeds | 13 | 13 | 74 |

|  | Carbohydrate (%) | Protein (%) | Fat (%) |
|---|---|---|---|
| **Grains and pseudograins** | | | |
| Amaranth | 69 | 14 | 17 |
| Brown rice, medium-grain | 85 | 8 | 7 |
| Buckwheat | 78 | 14 | 8 |
| Millet | 78 | 12 | 10 |
| Oats, rolled | 71 | 14 | 15 |
| Quinoa | 70 | 15 | 15 |
| Wheat, unsprouted | 82 | 14 | 4 |
| Wheat, sprouted | 81 | 14 | 5 |
| Wild rice | 81 | 16 | 3 |
| **Algae and grasses** | | | |
| Barley grass powder | 55 | 34 | 11 |
| Kelp | 77 | 13 | 10 |
| Nori | 44 | 50 | 6 |
| Spirulina | 24 | 58 | 18 |
| Wheatgrass powder | 55 | 34 | 11 |
| **Legumes** | | | |
| Alfalfa sprouts | 28 | 52 | 20 |
| Chickpeas | 65 | 21 | 14 |
| Green peas | 70 | 26 | 4 |
| Green peas, sprouted | 72 | 24 | 4 |
| Lentils, dry | 68 | 29 | 3 |
| Lentils, sprouted | 68 | 29 | 3 |
| Mung beans | 70 | 27 | 3 |
| Mung beans, sprouted | 63 | 33 | 4 |
| Peanuts, raw | 11 | 17 | 72 |
| **Animal foods (for comparison)** | | | |
| Beef, 80% lean | 0 | 29 | 71 |
| Chicken breast, skinless | 0 | 62 | 38 |
| Egg | 6 | 32 | 62 |
| Milk, 2% fat | 39 | 26 | 35 |
| Salmon, wild Alaskan | 0 | 73 | 27 |

## Grains and Pseudograins

What's the difference between a grain and a pseudograin? True grains are in the botanical family Poaceae, also known as the grass family. This includes wheat, rye, oats, rice, corn, and barley. We use the term pseudograin to refer to foods that have some nutritional similarities to grains, but are not actually in the botanical grain family. Three examples of pseudograins are buckwheat, quinoa, and amaranth. Buckwheat is in the knotweed family (Polygonaceae), whereas quinoa and amaranth are in the amaranth family (Amaranthaceae). The protein, gluten, and mineral content can differ significantly between true grains and pseudograins. Pseudograins are considered to be gluten-free, but we have observed that some very gluten-sensitive people may have trouble with them for various reasons.

### Algae and Grasses

If you're at all concerned about getting enough protein on a raw food diet (which we hope you aren't after reading chapter 4), including relatively small amounts of the algae shown in table 1.1 can provide a lot of protein. Spirulina is one of the lowest calorie sources of protein that I've seen. It's not botanically an alga; more specifically, it's classified as a type of cyanobacteria, which can employ photosynthesis like plants can. Kelp is a brown alga, and nori is a red alga.

Powdered dried grass is often a part of green food formulas commonly consumed by many raw-food enthusiasts, often along with some of the algae listed in table 1.1. Powdered grasses are primarily composed of carbohydrates but also contain a substantial amount of protein and are relatively low in fat.

### Legumes and Sprouts

Legumes, with the exception of peanuts, are low in fat and high in protein. They are frequently sprouted in a raw food diet, and alfalfa, lentil, and mung are popular types of legume sprouts.

## In Summary

Now that you have an overview of the carbohydrate, protein, and fat content of various foods, we'll delve more deeply into each of the individual macronutrients.

## CHAPTER 2

# Carbohydrates and Fiber

ALL WHOLE PLANT FOODS CONTAIN CARBOHYDRATES. Other than the simple carbohydrate lactose found in dairy products, animal foods contain little, if any, carbohydrates. The amount and types of carbohydrates in plant foods can differ substantially.

Carbohydrates can be categorized as monosaccharides, disaccharides, or polysaccharides according to the complexity of their molecular structure, ranging from simple to complex:

**Monosaccharide.** The simplest carbohydrates are known as monosaccharides; "mono" means one and "saccharide" means sugar. There are three different types of monosaccharides: glucose, fructose, and galactose. Glucose is the fuel of choice for most of the cells in the body, with the exception of heart muscle cells, which prefer to run on fat. The term blood sugar means blood glucose, so when someone is measuring their blood sugar, they're actually measuring the concentration of glucose in their blood. Fructose is similar in structure to glucose. Galactose is part of the sugar lactose found in animal milks. All three monosaccharides can be used to create energy.

Sweet fruits have notable amounts of fructose and in some cases glucose, but most do not contain galactose, other than in a few exceptions where there are extremely small amounts. Meat does not contain any monosaccharides, since animal flesh does not contain significant quantities of carbohydrate—only protein and fat. Meat may actually contain small amounts of carbohydrate in the form of glycogen, but considering the number of calories in this amount of carbohydrate, the amount is negligible in comparison to the amounts of fat and protein in meat. For example, nutrient databases list the carbohydrate content of meat as zero, which is true for all practical purposes.

**Disaccharide.** A disaccharide is a simple sugar consisting of two monosaccharides. There are three disaccharides: sucrose, maltose, and lactose. Sucrose is composed of one glucose molecule and one fructose molecule and can be found in many natural and processed foods, with one of the most prevalent forms being white table sugar. Maltose is composed of two glucose molecules and can be found as an ingredient in processed foods. Lactose is composed of one glucose molecule and one galactose molecule and, as was stated earlier, is the only sugar of animal origin.

**Table 2.1.** Monosaccharide and disaccharide content of select foods

| | Calories (kcal) | Glucose (g) | Fructose (g) | Galactose (g) | Sucrose (g) | Maltose (g) | Lactose (g) |
|---|---|---|---|---|---|---|---|
| **Sweet fruits** | | | | | | | |
| Apple, 1 medium (182 g) | 95 | 4.4 | 10.7 | 0 | 3.8 | 0 | 0 |
| Banana, 1 medium (118 g) | 105 | 5.9 | 5.7 | 0 | 2.8 | 0.01 | 0 |
| Blueberries, 1 c (148 g) | 84 | 7.2 | 7.4 | 0 | 0.2 | 0 | 0 |
| Dates, medjool, 1 pitted (24 g) | 66.5 | 8.1 | 7.7 | 0 | 0.1 | 0.1 | 0 |
| Strawberries, 1 c (166 g) | 53 | 3.3 | 4 | 0 | 0.8 | 0 | 0 |
| **Vegetables** | | | | | | | |
| Carrots, grated, 1 c (110 g) | 45 | 0.7 | 0.6 | 0 | 4 | 0 | 0 |
| Romaine lettuce, 1 lb, 6 oz (626 g) | 106 | 2.3 | 4.7 | 0 | 0 | 0 | 0 |
| Tomatoes, chopped, 1 c (180 g) | 32 | 2.3 | 2.5 | 0 | 0 | 0 | 0 |
| Yam, 4½ oz (130 g) | 112 | 1.3 | 0.9 | 0 | 3.3 | 0 | 0 |
| **Fats and oils** | | | | | | | |
| Almonds, ½ c (71.5 g) | 411 | 0.1 | 0.1 | 0.1 | 2.6 | 0.03 | 0 |
| Avocado, medium (201 g) | 322 | 0.7 | 0.2 | 0.2 | 0.1 | 0 | 0 |
| Coconut oil, unrefined, 1 Tbsp (14 g) | 120 | 0 | 0 | 0 | 0 | 0 | 0 |
| Olive oil, extra virgin, 1 Tbsp (13.5 g) | 119 | 0 | 0 | 0 | 0 | 0 | 0 |
| **Animal products** | | | | | | | |
| Beef, 80% lean, 4 oz (113.4 g) | 288 | 0 | 0 | 0 | 0 | 0 | 0 |
| Chicken breast, skinless, 4 oz (113.4 g) | 155 | 0 | 0 | 0 | 0 | 0 | 0 |
| Cow's milk, 2%, 1 c (244 g) | 122 | 0.02 | 0.02 | 0.5 | 0.02 | 0.02 | 11.28 |
| Salmon, pink, 4 oz (113.4 g) | 169 | 0 | 0 | 0 | 0 | 0 | 0 |

The sweet fruits in table 2.1 contain more sucrose than maltose and lactose, as sucrose is a combination of the monosaccharides fructose and glucose. Sucrose content can vary depending on the fruit, and a good example is the sucrose content of bananas compared to apples. Other than fruits, the foods listed in this table are not rich in disaccharides, since they're also not rich sources of simple carbohydrate. One exception is cow's milk, since dairy products are rich in lactose.

**Polysaccharide.** The carbohydrates found in vegetables (as well as grains and pseudograins) are more complex. A complex carbohydrate, or polysaccharide, is a series of monosaccharides linked together. Some polysaccharides provide calories, while others do not.

Starch, glycogen, and fiber are all examples of polysaccharides. Starch is the complex carbohydrate found in plants that provides us with usable energy, as it ultimately breaks down into monosaccharides. Starch is broken down by carbohydrate-digesting enzymes in the digestive tract to form the simple carbohydrate glucose, which can then be absorbed and utilized by the body. Glycogen is the storage form of carbohydrate in the human body and is retained in the liver and skeletal muscles. Fiber (also known as cellulose) is not broken down by digestive enzymes but passes through the digestive tract intact and doesn't directly provide us with energy. However, it has other benefits, such as helping to keep blood cholesterol at appropriate levels and maintaining bowel regularity.

Sweet fruits are naturally low in starch, since most of the carbohydrates they contain are monosaccharides and disaccharides. Carrots and yams are much higher in starch, since most of the carbohydrates they contain are polysaccharides. Animal foods do not contain complex carbohydrates.

## Fiber's Role as a Prebiotic

Most types of fiber are composed of glucose molecules; however, one type of fiber, inulin, is composed of fructose molecules. As with all fiber, inulin is not broken down by digestive enzymes, but it can be digested by beneficial intestinal bacteria. Because it can provide food for those helpful bacteria (known as probiotics), inulin is referred to as a prebiotic.

Fructooligosaccharides (FOS) are other types of fiber similar to inulin that are composed of fructose molecules. Fructooligosaccharides generally have between two and ten fructose molecules linked together, whereas inulins contain over ten fructose molecules and are considered to be polysaccharides. Because FOS molecules are not as long as inulin molecules, they're classified as oligosaccharides (few sugars). A *Journal of Nutrition* study reported that both FOS and inulin can be food sources for probiotics and that they occur naturally in more than 36,000 plant species in varying amounts, as shown in table 2.2 on the next page.

**Table 2.2.** The inulin and FOS content of select foods*

| Food | Inulin content (mg/g fresh plant weight) | FOS content (mg/g fresh plant weight) |
|---|---|---|
| Banana, ripe | 3–7 | 2.0 |
| Garlic bulb | 90–160 | 3.9 |
| Jerusalem artichoke or sunchoke (tuber) | 140–190 | 58.4 |
| Onion bulb | 20–60 | 3.1 |
| Leek bulb | 30–100 | 0.9 |
| Rye | 5–10 | 3.8 |
| Barley | 5–15 | 1.7 |

* Other foods high in inulin are artichoke hearts, burdock root, chicory root, dandelion leaves, and yacon root (a South American tuber similar in flavor to jicama).

*Sources:* Data from Campbell et al. (1997); Van Loo et al. (1995).

Fructooligosaccharides tend to have a mildly sweet taste, while fructose is notably sweeter. If you've ever tasted raw sunchokes (Jerusalem artichokes), yacon root, or jicama, you might have noticed the mild, sweet flavor that comes from the fructooligosaccharides or inulin they contain. Contrast this to high-fructose foods that have an intensely sweet flavor, such as oranges, apples, and mangoes.

## Carbohydrate Misconceptions

Carbohydrates are often lumped together into one group without regard for the important differences that exist among individual carbohydrate-rich foods. Not all carbohydrates are created equal. Another point to note is that nearly all foods contain carbohydrates, with the exceptions of meat, oil, or processed foods in which the carbohydrates have been removed.

### Carbohydrate Contribution to Obesity

There are many causes of overweight and obesity, with the most common being the overconsumption of calories. When excess calories are consumed, the body stores carbohydrate, fat, and protein as body fat.

Many processed carbohydrate-rich foods are also high in added fat and in some cases contain more fat than carbohydrate. (See table 2.3.) Since the body will generally use carbohydrate as fuel before it uses fat, the fat in these foods is often converted to body fat. Depending on how many excess calories are consumed, carbohydrate and protein can also be converted to body fat. So, are the carbohydrates in these foods really the issue, or could it be the fat they contain?

**Table 2.3.** Carbohydrate-rich processed foods

|  | Carbohydrate (%) | Fat (%) | Protein (%) |
|---|---|---|---|
| Potato chips | 35 | 60 | 5 |
| Croissant | 45 | 47 | 8 |
| Glazed doughnut | 46 | 49 | 5 |
| Candy bar | 49 | 45 | 6 |
| French fries | 49 | 46 | 5 |
| Blueberry muffin | 57 | 37 | 6 |
| White bread | 77 | 10 | 13 |
| Bagel, plain | 80 | 5 | 15 |

## The Effect of Carbohydrates on Blood Sugar

Most carbohydrates ultimately break down into the simple carbohydrate glucose. Generally, if glucose is released and absorbed into the bloodstream quickly, blood glucose levels increase, and there will be a corresponding increase in the production of insulin, the hormone responsible for escorting glucose out of the blood and into the cells, such as muscle cells. If this glucose is not used for the creation of energy, it may turn into fat. So one may say that insulin is responsible for providing glucose to cells to meet their energy needs; however, if the cells don't have a current need for energy, insulin is responsible for telling the body to make and store fat in order to store that energy for later use.

It's not unusual to think that all carbohydrates raise blood glucose because of their sugar content. To measure this more accurately, a system called the glycemic index (GI) was created by David Jenkins, MD, and his colleagues at the University of Toronto to determine how much each gram of total carbohydrate (less any fiber) in a food raises blood sugar, compared to the increase caused by eating pure glucose by itself. The recent work of researchers at the University of Sydney has provided invaluable data on the glycemic index and glycemic load values of numerous popularly consumed foods, as we will see shortly. For the most part, foods with a high ranking on the glycemic index cause a higher rise in blood glucose. Foods that score lower on the GI rating system produce a comparatively slower rise in blood sugar and insulin levels. Foods are ranked according to this value as being low, moderate, and high glycemic.

|  | Low | Moderate | High |
|---|---|---|---|
| Glycemic Index | ≤55 | 56–69 | 70–100+ |

Fructose is low on the glycemic index even though it's a simple carbohydrate. Sucrose is composed of equal amounts of glucose and fructose, so it makes sense that the glycemic index of sucrose is somewhere between glucose and fructose. In general, the higher the glucose and sucrose content of a food, the higher the glycemic index.

| Simple Carbohydrate | Glycemic Index |
|---|---|
| Fructose | 15 ± 4 |
| Glucose | 103 ± 3 |
| Sucrose | 65 ± 4 |

The symbol "±" means plus or minus, showing the glycemic range of the food in question. For example, fructose has a glycemic range of 11 to 19.

Many sweet fruits are surprisingly low on the glycemic index, while others are higher, as shown in table 2.4. In general, fruits with a greater glucose and sucrose content tend to be higher on the glycemic index than fruits with a greater fructose or fiber content, or both. This is an important point, because all too often fruits, especially sweet fruits, are needlessly avoided because people think they are high glycemic.

**Table 2.4.** The glycemic index values of selected fruits

| Food | Glycemic index (glucose = 100) |
|---|---|
| Cherries | 22 |
| Grapefruit | 25 |
| Apple | 36 ± 2 |
| Pear | 38 ± 2 |
| Strawberries | 40 ± 7 |
| Peach | 42 ± 14 |
| Grapes | 46 ± 3 |
| Banana | 51 ± 3 |
| Mango | 51 ± 5 |
| Pineapple | 59 ± 8 |
| Figs, dried | 61 ± 6 |
| Raisins | 64 ± 11 |
| Watermelon | 76 ± 4 |

Students often ask about the GI for dates. A 2011 study published in the *Nutrition Journal* reported that average GI values were 46 for bo ma'an dates and 55 for khalas dates in nondiabetic participants. An earlier study, published in 2002 in the *Saudi Medical Journal*, found the mean GIs for three types of dates to be 31 for bo ma'an, 36 for khalas, and 50 for barhi dates. The differences in these numbers may be due to a variety of factors, such as the natural variation between samples and biochemical differences between study volunteers. Both studies indicate that these dates are in the low to low-moderate GI range. I have yet to find a reliable GI for medjool dates.

I've heard people say they won't eat carrots because of the perceived sugar content and a fear that carrots will raise blood sugar. However, table 2.5 shows that processed foods containing carbohydrates tend to be notably higher on the glycemic index than high-carbohydrate whole foods. Generally, the greater the processing, the higher the glycemic index. Cooking will also increase the glycemic index of whole foods, because it may increase the availability of glucose in some foods (but sometimes only slightly). Greens and other foods that are naturally low in glucose and fructose are usually not listed on glycemic index charts.

**Table 2.5.** The glycemic index of selected whole foods and processed foods

| Food | Glycemic index (glucose = 100) |
| --- | --- |
| Carrots, raw | 16 |
| Chickpeas | 28 ± 9 |
| Lentils | 32 ± 5 |
| Yam | 37 ± 8 |
| Carrots, boiled | 39 ± 4 |
| Specialty grain bread | 53 ± 2 |
| Brown rice | 55 ± 5 |
| Soft drink | 59 ± 3 |
| Honey | 61 ± 3 |
| Croissant | 67 |
| Pancakes | 67 ± 5 |
| Oatmeal | 69 |
| Bagel, white | 72 |
| White rice | 73 ± 4 (low GI varieties also identified) |
| White wheat bread | 75 ± 2 |
| Jelly beans | 78 ± 2 |
| Cornflakes | 81 ± 6 |

## Glycemic Load Versus Glycemic Index

As stated above, the glycemic index (GI) measures the effect of the carbohydrate in a food on blood sugar levels. Another measurement, the glycemic load (GL), builds upon the glycemic index by taking the quantity of carbohydrate consumed into account as well. The official definition of glycemic load is the quantity of carbohydrate consumed multiplied by the glycemic index of the carbohydrate consumed, divided by 100. The equation looks like this:

$$\text{Glycemic load (GL)} = \frac{\text{Carbohydrate content (g) x Glycemic index (GI)}}{100}$$

In general, a food with a low glycemic index tends to create a lower glycemic load than the same quantity of food with a higher glycemic index. However, there are many exceptions to this rule. A great example is watermelon, which is notorious for its high glycemic index. Watermelon is aptly named because of its high water content, which dilutes the carbohydrate content. Therefore, the glycemic load of a meal high in watermelon is low despite the high glycemic index, as the quantity of carbohydrate consumed does not tend to be high. By the time someone is full of watermelon, they've

**Table 2.6.** The glycemic load* of selected fruits

| Serving size | Glycemic index | Available carbohydrate content (g) | Glycemic load per serving |
|---|---|---|---|
| Cherries, 1 c (154 g) | 22 | 24.7 | 5 |
| Grapefruit, whole (236 g) | 25 | 21.5 | 5 |
| Apple, medium (182 g) | 36 | 25.1 | 9 |
| Pear, medium (178 g) | 38 | 27.5 | 10 |
| Strawberries, 1 c sliced (166 g) | 40 | 12.8 | 5 |
| Peach, medium (150 g) | 42 | 14.3 | 6 |
| Grapes, 1 c (151 g) | 46 | 27.3 | 13 |
| Banana, medium (118 g) | 51 | 27.0 | 14 |
| Mango, whole (207 g) | 51 | 35.2 | 18 |
| Pineapple, 1 c chunks (165 g) | 59 | 21.7 | 13 |
| Figs, 5 fresh (255 g) | 61 | 46.7 | 28 |
| Raisins, ½ c unpacked (73 g) | 64 | 57.4 | 37 |
| Watermelon, 1 c diced (152 g) | 76 | 11.5 | 9 |

* Glycemic load values calculated from glycemic index values found in Foster-Powell et al.

eaten much more water than carbohydrate, which keeps the quantity of carbohydrates consumed low. Raisins, on the other hand, have a similar glycemic index to watermelon but can create a much higher glycemic load, given that raisins have a low water content and the carbohydrates they contain are therefore much more concentrated. By the time someone gets full from eating raisins, the quantity of carbohydrates they've consumed can be very large. A particular weight or volume of raisins contains much more carbohydrate than a similar amount of watermelon.

Like the glycemic index, foods are rated low, moderate, or high.

|  | Low | Moderate | High |
|---|---|---|---|
| Glycemic Load | ≤10 | 11–19 | ≥20 |

It's not surprising that highly processed foods have higher glycemic loads than less processed or unprocessed foods. Oatmeal and brown rice, which are generally cooked in water, both have moderate glycemic index values and are borderline low to moderate in glycemic load. In contrast, more concentrated, processed carbohydrate-rich foods, such as croissants and pancakes that have a similar GI to oatmeal, can create a much higher glycemic load. The lower water content and lower fiber content of croissants and pancakes makes them more concentrated than oatmeal and brown rice. This generally leads to greater quantities of carbohydrates consumed in a given meal. Fiber has an additional role in the glycemic index component of the glycemic load, in that it lowers the glycemic index of a food. It should not be surprising then that high-fiber multigrain bread has a lower glycemic load than low-fiber white bread, and that the water- and fiber-rich whole foods in table 2.7 on the next page (including raw and cooked carrots, cooked chickpeas, cooked lentils, and baked yam) have a lower glycemic load per serving than the more concentrated foods in that table.

Question: How many cups of grated raw carrots would you have to eat to get the equivalent glycemic load of one bagel? Answer: approximately 20 cups. Both raw and cooked carrots are low on the glycemic index and have low glycemic loads, and the same is true for many sweet fruits! For example, it would take nearly three medium bananas or 4½ cups of watermelon to equal the glycemic load of that same bagel. Considering their glycemic index and glycemic load, these fruits don't have to be avoided. It's true that these foods can affect insulin levels, but so too can low-carbohydrate foods, such as cuts of meat. Due to the complexity of this topic, we further discuss the effect of foods on insulin levels in our series of Science of Raw Food Nutrition classes.

**Table 2.7.** The glycemic load* of selected whole foods and processed foods

| Serving size | Glycemic index | Available carbohydrate content (g) | Glycemic load per serving |
|---|---|---|---|
| Carrots, raw, 1 c grated (110 g) | 16 | 10.5 | 2 |
| Chickpeas, cooked, ½ c (82 g) | 28 | 22.5 | 6 |
| Lentils, cooked, ½ c (99 g) | 32 | 19.9 | 6 |
| Yam, baked, 4 oz (114 g) | 37 | 23.6 | 8 |
| Carrots, boiled, 1 c sliced (156 g) | 39 | 12.8 | 5 |
| Specialty grain bread, 2 slices (52 g) | 53 | 22.5 | 12 |
| Brown rice, long-grain, cooked, ½ c (98 g) | 55 | 22.4 | 12 |
| Cola soft drink, 2 c (492 g) | 59 | 53.3 | 31 |
| Honey, 1 Tbsp (21 g) | 61 | 17.3 | 11 |
| Croissant, 2 oz (57 g) | 67 | 26.1 | 17 |
| Pancakes, about 4 medium (53 g) | 67 | 31.8 | 21 |
| Oatmeal, ½ c cooked (117 g) | 69 | 14 | 10 |
| Bagel, white, 3½ oz (105 g) | 72 | 56.1 | 40 |
| White rice, long-grain, cooked, ½ c (79 g) | 73 | 22.3 | 16 |
| White bread, 2 slices (50 g) | 75 | 25.3 | 19 |
| Jelly beans, 10 large (28 g) | 78 | 26.2 | 20 |
| Cornflakes, 1 c dry (28 g) | 81 | 24.4 | 20 |

* Glycemic load values calculated from glycemic index values found in Foster-Powell et al.

## The Difference Between Fructose and High-Fructose Corn Syrup

On occasion, I've heard people equate fructose to high-fructose corn syrup, but these two substances have a very different composition and effect on blood sugar. Fructose is a monosaccharide; however, high-fructose corn syrup is a combination of fructose and glucose. There are also several types of high-fructose corn syrup created by food companies and used in a variety of processed food products. One of the more popular forms of high-fructose corn syrup is HFCS 55, which is composed of approximately 55 percent fructose and 45 percent glucose.

**Table 2.8.** The glycemic index of HFCS 55 compared to simple carbohydrates

|  | Glycemic index (Glucose = 100) |
|---|---|
| Glucose | 103 ± 3 |
| Sucrose | 65 ± 4 |
| High-fructose corn syrup (HFCS 55) | 62 |
| Fructose | 15 ± 4 |

Fructose is much lower on the glycemic index than glucose, sucrose, and high-fructose corn syrup. It makes sense that sucrose and high-fructose corn syrup have similar glycemic index values, since sucrose is composed of 50 percent glucose and 50 percent fructose. It also makes sense that both sucrose and high-fructose corn syrup would have glycemic index values in between glucose and fructose, since both sucrose and high-fructose corn syrup are composed of some combination of both glucose and fructose. Fructose has much less of an effect on blood sugar than high-fructose corn syrup.

## Carbohydrates, the Whole Picture

Carbohydrate-rich whole foods, such as fruits and vegetables, make a significant contribution to our energy needs, and one of the great benefits of a raw diet is the freedom to enjoy these whole-food carbohydrates without worry. Understanding the concepts of glycemic index and glycemic load can help people make educated decisions about food choices by elucidating the differences between whole-food and processed carbohydrates, and especially clarifying the frequent misunderstandings about the actual glycemic index values of fruit.

CHAPTER 3

# Fat

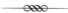

ENERGY IS STORED IN THE BODY PRIMARILY AS FAT. When dietary fat is consumed in excess of the body's needs, it's stored in fat cells for later use as a potential source of energy. When protein or carbohydrates are consumed in excess of the body's needs, they're converted into fat, which is also stored in fat cells. Fat is also used by the body to cushion organs, affect the levels and functioning of different types of hormones, regulate inflammatory processes, and maintain cell membrane integrity.

Dietary fats can be divided into two major categories: saturated and unsaturated. The key difference between saturated and unsaturated fats has to do with the presence of double bonds in their structure. Saturated fats don't contain double bonds, while unsaturated fats do contain them. Saturated fats are stiff and rigid, don't conduct electrical activity, and are more chemically stable. In contrast, unsaturated fats are flexible and fluid, conduct electrical activity, and are less chemically stable.

The greater the number of double bonds in an unsaturated fat, the more susceptible it is to degradation and rancidity (also known as oxidation or free radical damage). A free radical is a molecule with a missing electron that can cause damage to body structures. Cell membranes are primarily made from a mixture of fats and are a great example of a body structure that utilizes the characteristics of saturated and unsaturated fats to function properly. The unsaturated fats found in cell membranes are particularly susceptible to free radical damage. Fortunately, a diet rich in fruits and vegetables contains a variety of antioxidants to protect unsaturated fats from this type of damage.

The building blocks of fats are known as fatty acids. The length of the fatty acid chain, as well as the number and location of double bonds, if any, determines the type of fat, such as the following:

**Saturated fat.** Saturated fatty acids have no double bonds. An example is lauric acid, found in coconut oil.

**Monounsaturated fat.** Monounsaturated fatty acids contain one double bond. An example is oleic acid, the principle fat found in olive oil.

**Polyunsaturated fat.** Polyunsaturated fatty acids contain more than one double bond. An example is alpha-linolenic acid (ALA), the principle fat found in flaxseeds and chia seeds.

Two polyunsaturated fatty acids are considered to be essential, because the body needs these fats in order to function properly but does not make them. They must be obtained from sources outside the body. These two are alpha-linolenic acid (ALA), an omega-3 fat, and linoleic acid (LA), an omega-6 fat.

## The Essential Fatty Acids

Two polyunsaturated fats are known as essential fats:
• alpha-linolenic acid (ALA), an omega-3 fat
• linoleic acid (LA), an omega-6 fat

ALA is the building block, or parent fatty acid, for the other members of the omega-3 family. Those that play very important roles in the body are known as eicosapentaenoic acid (EPA) and docosahexaenoic acid (DHA). EPA is well known for its role in reducing inflammation. DHA allows metabolically active tissues, such as the brain, retina of the eye, adrenals, and testes, to function properly. It plays important roles in cell membranes by helping the cells to function properly and allows the hormones that affect these cells to direct cellular functions most effectively and appropriately.

DHA contains six double bonds, more than any other commonly examined fat of nutritional significance in the body. On the one hand, these double bonds allow DHA to conduct the electrical activity needed for the metabolically active tissues mentioned previously, while on the other hand these same double bonds make DHA very susceptible to oxidation. Therefore, DHA is usually only made by organisms when they need it or when metabolic conditions are favorable.

EPA contains five double bonds, which gives it many of the same attributes as DHA, particularly that it stays fluid and flexible at very cold temperatures. EPA and DHA, not surprisingly, are found in the greatest abundance in organisms that live in cold water. The primary source of EPA and DHA in the ocean food chain is certain EPA- and DHA-containing algae. Fish and other marine animals obtain these fats when they eat these algae, when they eat fish that have eaten the algae, and so on up the food chain. The algae can also be consumed in the human diet as a direct source of these omega-3 fats.

Linoleic acid (LA) is the building block, or parent fatty acid, for the other members of the omega-6 family. Those that play very important roles in the body are known as di-homo-gamma-linolenic acid (DGLA) and arachidonic acid (AA). AA is well known for its role in promoting inflammation. Although inflammation is an important part of the healing process, too much prolonged inflammation can lead to tissue damage, and getting the proper balance between omega-6 fats and omega-3 fats plays a significant role in regulating inflammation. Fats in the omega-3 family are generally anti-inflammatory, whereas fats in the omega-6 family are generally pro-inflammatory.

The research of Artemis Simopoulos, James Greenberg, and Gerry Schwalfenberg suggests that up until several hundred years ago humans may have consumed omega-6 fats and omega-3 fats in almost equal amounts, a ratio of 1:1 to 1.5:1. It's estimated that in the current Western diet, this ratio is in the range of 15:1, and even as high as 25:1. Clinical research has shown that ratios between 2.5:1 and 5:1 create the best outcomes for a variety of health challenges, while ratios of 10:1 have shown less favorable outcomes. A lower omega-6 to omega-3 ratio is thought of as more desirable for reducing risk for certain chronic diseases found in Western society. This is not surprising, since many chronic diseases are thought to have an inflammatory component.

Linoleic acid is particularly abundant in the refined vegetable oils consumed in great quantity in Western diets. Although alpha-linolenic acid can be challenging to find, even on a standard omnivorous Western diet, it's present in leafy greens consumed in significant quantities, as well as flaxseeds, chia seeds, hemp seeds, and a few other sources.

## Maintaining a Good Omega-6 to Omega-3 Balance

Table 3.1 on the next page shows a comparison of samples of plant and animal sources of unsaturated fatty acids, along with the ratio between omega-6 and omega-3 fats in each food. Chia seeds and flaxseeds are especially strong sources of the omega-3 fat alpha-linolenic acid. Not surprisingly, chia seeds and flaxseeds both have the lowest omega-6 to omega-3 ratios of the nuts and seeds listed, with the vegetables in this table having a similar ratio.

Hemp seeds and English walnuts are considered to be good sources of ALA, but they have more omega-6 than omega-3 fats. Sacha inchi seeds and oil have roughly equal amounts of omega-6 and omega-3 fats. Chia seeds and flaxseeds, with three and four times more omega-3 than omega-6 fats, respectively, are best able to create a healthy ratio by offsetting the omega-6 content of other foods that are commonly consumed in excess relative to omega-3s. When omega-6 foods are not consumed in excess, hemp seeds and walnuts may be perfectly suitable, as long as the overall omega-6 to omega-3 ratio falls within the healthy ranges listed above.

Most leafy greens and vegetables, such as those found in table 3.1, have favorable omega-6 to omega-3 ratios. Note that the actual amount of ALA that vegetables contain per serving is much smaller than that of chia seeds and flaxseeds, since leafy greens and other vegetables contain much less fat than these foods. However, large vegetable salads containing significant amounts of leafy greens (such as the raw salad on the facing page) as well as green smoothies can provide a notable amount of ALA.

**Table 3.1.** A comparison of selected foods with a desirable ratio of omega-3 fats

| Food | omega-6 fat (%) | omega-3 fat (%) | omega-6: omega-3 ratio |
|---|---|---|---|
| **Fruits** | | | |
| Banana | 14 | 8 | 1.8:1 |
| Strawberries | 30 | 22 | 1.4:1 |
| **Vegetables** | | | |
| Cauliflower | 11 | 38 | 1:3 |
| Kale | 20 | 26 | 1:1.3 |
| Lettuce, romaine | 16 | 38 | 1:2.5 |
| Lettuce, green leaf | 16 | 39 | 1:2.5 |
| Zucchini | 16 | 26 | 1:2 |
| **Nuts, seeds, and oils** | | | |
| Chia seeds | 19 | 57 | 1:3 |
| Flax oil | 13 | 53 | 1:4 |
| Flaxseeds | 14 | 54 | 1:4 |
| Hemp seeds | 60 | 18 | 3.3:1 |
| Walnuts, English | 58 | 14 | 4:1 |
| *Sacha inchi seeds | 34–50 | 36–44 | 1.1:1 |
| *Sacha inchi oil | 34–36 | 45–50 | 1:1.4 |
| **Fish (for comparison)** | | | |
| Fish oil, salmon | 2 | 32 | 1:14.6 |
| Salmon, farmed Atlantic | 7 | 32 | 1:3 |
| Salmon, wild Pacific | 3 | 35 | 1:12.5 |

* Sources: Data from Fanali et al. (2011); Follegatti-Romero et al. (2009); Hamaker et al. (1992); Maurer et al. (2012)

The current adequate intake (AI) for ALA is 1.6 grams. However, in 2005 Harvard researcher Dariush Mozaffarian stated that most evidence suggests an intake of 2 to 3 grams may be even more beneficial. At this time, there is no Dietary Reference Intake (DRI) for DHA and EPA, but the European Food Safety Authority suggests a collective intake of 250–500 milligrams per day for adults.

It may be a challenge to find omega-3 fats in significant amounts on a raw food diet, unless you're familiar with reliable sources. On the other hand, omega-6 fats are easily found, given that they are present in so many

### Raw Salad and Dressing Ingredients

Here are the ingredients for a typical salad eaten by people following a raw diet, along with the amount of omega fatty acids and their ratio.

### Salad

4 cups (188 g) chopped romaine lettuce
4 cups (99 g) chopped dandelion greens
1 cup (180 g) chopped tomatoes
1 cup (110 g) grated carrots
1 cup (104 g) chopped cucumber
½ cup (21.2 g) chopped fresh basil

### Salad Dressing

1 cup (149 g) chopped red bell pepper
1 cup (124 g) chopped zucchini
¼ cup (61 g) fresh-squeezed lemon juice
2 tablespoons (20 g) chia seeds
1 tablespoon (9 g) almonds
1 tablespoon (9 g) unhulled sesame seeds

Percentage of fat content as omega-6 and omega-3 fats:
• omega-6 fat: 30 percent (5 g)
• omega-3 fat: 22 percent (4 g)
• omega-6:omega-3 ratio = 1.25:1

The omega-6 to omega-3 ratio in this salad is favorable, despite the inclusion of sesame seeds, which are high in omega-6s, in the dressing. The omega-3 content of the leafy greens and especially the chia seeds helps to offset the omega-6 fats in sesame seeds, almonds, and other foods.

---

foods in notable amounts. Table 3.2 on page 26 shows a selection of common foods that are high in omega-6 fats.

It's important to note that the foods listed in this table are not good sources of omega-3 fats. I included these foods because many of them are popular in the raw-food community, with the exception of these particular oils and animal foods, which are common in the standard Western diet. If you're trying to optimize your omega-6 to omega-3 ratio, you may want to consider the significant omega-6 content of the foods and oils in table 3.2.

**Table 3.2.** A comparison of selected foods high in omega-6 fats

| Food | omega-6 (%) | omega-3 fat (%) | omega-6: omega-3 ratio |
|---|---|---|---|
| **Grains and pseudograins** | | | |
| Buckwheat | 28 | 2 | 12:1 |
| Corn | 45 | 2 | 31.5:1 |
| Quinoa | 49 | 5 | 11.5:1 |
| Rice, brown | 34 | 2 | 22.5:1 |
| Wheat, red winter | 39 | 2 | 19.3:1 |
| **Oils** | | | |
| Corn oil | 54 | 1.1 | 49:1 |
| Cottonseed oil | 52 | 0.2 | 260:1 |
| Safflower oil | 75 | 0 | - |
| Soy oil | 51 | 7 | 7.3:1 |
| Sunflower oil | 40 | 0.2 | 200:1 |
| **Seeds** | | | |
| Poppy seeds | 68 | 1 | 79:1 |
| Pumpkin seeds | 42 | 0.25 | 168:1 |
| Sesame seeds | 43 | 0.12 | 57:1 |
| Sunflower seeds | 45 | 0.12 | 37:1 |
| **Animal foods (for comparison)** | | | |
| Beef, 80% lean | 2 | 0.3 | 7:1 |
| Chicken breast, skinless | 21 | 2 | 11:1 |
| Egg | 13 | 0.7 | 19:1 |
| Cow's milk, 2% fat | 3 | 0.4 | 8:1 |

## Foods High in Omega-9 Fats

Omega-9 fats are not essential fatty acids. Many of the high-fat plant foods consumed by raw-food enthusiasts, such as almonds, avocados, cashews, macadamia nuts, olives, and olive oil, are high in the omega-9 fat oleic acid. Table 3.3 compares these foods and also gives their omega-6:omega-3 ratios.

These foods are not rich sources of omega-3 fats. This doesn't necessarily mean they're unhealthful or should be avoided; they're just not going to contribute meaningful amounts of omega-3 fats to your diet. You may also have noticed, particularly with almonds, Brazil nuts, and cashews, that even though their most abundant fat is omega-9, they also have a considerable amount of omega-6. Although to a lesser degree than foods that contain greater amounts of omega-6s, the net effect of eating these foods is pro-inflammatory. The best way to keep inflammation in check is to keep the consumption of these foods at low to moderate levels.

**Table 3.3.** A comparison of selected foods high in omega-9 fats

| Food | omega-6 (%) | omega-3 (%) | omega-9 (%) | omega-6: omega-3 ratio |
|------|-------------|-------------|-------------|------------------------|
| Almonds | 25 | 0.01 | 63 | 1,824:1 |
| Avocado, California | 10 | 0.7 | 64 | 14:1 |
| Brazil nuts | 31 | 0.03 | 37 | 1,033:1 |
| Cashews | 18 | 0.14 | 54 | 129:1 |
| Macadamia nuts | 1.7 | 0.3 | 78 | 16:1 |
| Olives, black | 8 | 0.6 | 74 | 13:1 |
| Olive oil | 10 | 0.7 | 73 | 14:1 |

## Saturated Fats and Their Sources

People most often associate saturated fat with animal foods, but a number of plant foods also contain them. Saturated fats are classified according to the length of their central carbon chains. The longer the saturated fat molecule, the higher the temperature needed to melt it (known as the melting point).

**Short-chain saturated fats (SCSFs).** These fats are six or fewer carbons in length and include acetic acid, found in vinegar, which is two carbons in length. Vinegar is obviously liquid at room temperature, while longer-chain saturated fats tend to be solid at room temperature.

**Medium-chain saturated fats (MCSFs).** These fats are between six and twelve carbons long and include lauric acid, found in coconut oil. The melting point of pure lauric acid is 109.9 degrees F (43.3 degrees C). The medium-chain saturated fats with shorter carbon chains melt at lower temperatures. Coconut oil is made up of a combination of medium-chain saturated fats (as well as some unsaturated fats) and has an overall melting point of 75 to 80 degrees F (24 to 27 degrees C).

**Long-chain saturated fats (LCSFs).** These fats have more than twelve carbons; very long-chain saturated fats (VLCSFs), those found most frequently in animal foods, have more than eighteen carbons. Foods containing LCSFs include palmitic acid, found in palm kernel oil, and stearic acid, generally found in animal foods. Cocoa butter contains both palmitic and steric acids. Cocoa and cacao butter melt at a much higher temperature than coconut oil, at 85.3 to 95 degrees F (29.6 to 35 degrees C).

**Table 3.4.** A comparison of foods high in saturated fats

| Food | omega-6 (%) | omega-3 (%) | omega-9 (%) | saturated (%) | omega-6: omega-3 ratio |
|---|---|---|---|---|---|
| Beef, grass fed | 3 | 0.5 | 38 | 42 | 6.25:1 |
| Beef, ground, 80% lean | 2 | 0.3 | 44 | 38 | 7:1 |
| Bison, grass fed | 4 | 0.5 | 38 | 40 | 7.6:1 |
| Butter | 3.3 | 0.38 | 26 | 63 | 9:1 |
| Cocoa butter | 2.8 | 0.01 | 33 | 60 | 280:1 |
| Coconut meat, mature | 1 | 0 | 4 | 89 | - |
| Coconut oil | 2 | 0 | 6 | 87 | - |
| Turkey, meat and skin | 22 | 1.4 | 36 | 28 | 16:1 |

None of these foods are significant sources of omega-3 fats. Although some of their omega-6 to omega-3 ratios are not too far out of range, their overall omega-3 content is very low and their saturated fat content is high. However, not all saturated fats are created equal. The Nurses' Health Study found that longer-chain saturated fats, such as those found primarily in animal foods, are more associated with increased risk for coronary artery disease than the shorter-chain saturated fats, such as those found in coconut oil. In addition, study participants consuming the highest ratio of unsaturated to saturated fats had lower risk for coronary artery disease when compared to study participants with lower ratios.

## Summary of Fat Balance on a Raw Diet

I've seen raw food menus with unfavorable omega-6 to omega-3 ratios and low ALA content when the menus contain notable amounts of olive oil and coconut oil, are high in omega-6 nuts and seeds, and have comparatively few omega-3 sources. (See more information on pages 148–152.) One way that I get more omega-3 fats into my diet is to add chia seeds to my evening salad dressing, eat plenty of vegetables (especially leafy greens) and fruits, and de-emphasize high omega-6 nuts and seeds overall. I still enjoy my sesame seeds and tahini—just not in large amounts—and I consume oil only once in a blue moon, such as in a restaurant meal. I choose to obtain my calories from whole foods, rather than oil.

# CHAPTER 4
# Protein

⎯⎯⎯∞∞∞⎯⎯⎯

"WHERE DO YOU GET YOUR PROTEIN?" is the most commonly asked question regarding vegetarian, vegan, and raw food nutrition. This question invariably comes up in any discussion of plant-based nutrition involving those new to the idea of eating a diet that doesn't include animal foods. Even people who have studied nutrition, plant-based or otherwise, for many years are often equally concerned and confused about obtaining this important macronutrient.

In this chapter, we'll go through a simple yet thorough exercise that will allow you to see just how easy it can be to get enough protein on a raw vegan diet. First, however, I'll lay a little bit of groundwork in order to help you make the most sense of the information that will answer this omnipresent, persistent, and inescapable question.

## Amino Acids

The building blocks of protein are 20 to 22 organic acids known as the standard amino acids, which we'll simply refer to as amino acids. When amino acids are assembled together in various combinations, different types of proteins are formed. This includes proteins that make up the structural components of our bodies, such as muscles, bones, skin, hair, nails, collagen, and parts of cells. Other proteins are used to create enzymes, hormones, antibodies, and neurotransmitters. All these proteins are essential for growth, repair, and good health.

In order for the body to manufacture proteins, all the amino acids must be available. Each specific protein does not necessarily use every one of the amino acids in its structure, just as each word or paragraph does not necessarily use each of the 26 letters in the English alphabet. However, if any one of the amino acids is in short supply, there will be at least some proteins that cannot be formed, and various structures and functional aspects of body systems will suffer.

Some of the amino acids can be made by the body, while the remainder cannot. Those that can be made by the body are known as the nonessential amino acids, while those that the body cannot make are known as the essential amino acids. It's "essential" to obtain the essential amino acids from an outside source, most preferably from foods in the diet.

## Recommended Protein Intakes

In 2007 the World Health Organization (WHO) published a 265-page report called "Protein and Amino Acid Requirements in Human Nutrition." This report examined protein and amino acid research studies from all over the world in order to come up with the WHO's most recent set of recommendations. Previous reports were published in 1991, 1985, and 1973.

As one might expect, the studies didn't all come to the exact same conclusion, even though they were trying to answer the same questions. When considering recommendations for the essential amino acid lysine, for example, studies ranged from recommendations of 17 to 30 milligrams of lysine for each kilogram of body weight, with 23 mg/kg being "the most secure value." The official WHO recommendation for lysine is listed as 30 mg/kg. As the WHO report states: "The estimates obtained are approximate and probably represent conservative overestimates, rather than underestimates, of the true values." In other words, the recommendations have a tendency to be on the high side, because WHO scientists want to be sure everyone's needs are covered.

The 2007 WHO protein recommendations are based on body weight, as people vary substantially in size and weight. For example, the protein needs of a male bodybuilder who consumes 4,000 calories per day may not be relevant for a less active, petite female who needs to consume only 1,600 calories per day to maintain her weight.

Total protein intake is the sum of all the amino acids consumed from the diet, essential and nonessential alike. The 2007 WHO recommendation for total protein intake is 0.8 grams of protein per kilogram of body weight. This recommendation is estimated to cover 97.5 percent of the human population's needs.

To calculate total protein recommendations for an individual, convert pounds of body weight into kilograms by dividing the weight in pounds by 2.2. Then multiply the weight in kilograms by 0.8, as shown in table 4.1. To compare this to the amount of total protein you consume daily, add up all the protein from all the foods you eat each day. Nutrient analysis software can come in very handy for this. All else being equal, the more calories you eat from whole natural foods, the higher your protein intake will be.

## WHO 2007 Essential Amino Acid Recommendations

Table 4.2 shows how much of each essential amino acid is recommended per kilogram of body weight, according to the most recent WHO report. Multiplying the recommendations per kilogram by 68 for someone weighing 68 kilograms (150 lbs) and then converting milligrams to grams results in the amount of each essential amino acid recommended by the WHO for someone of this weight.

**Table 4.1.** Calculating total protein recommendations based on body weight

| Weight in pounds | Converted to kilograms | Total protein recommended |
|---|---|---|
| 120 | 120 / 2.2 = 55 | 55 kg x 0.8 = 44 g |
| 150 | 150 / 2.2 = 68 | 68 kg x 0.8 = 54 g |
| 180 | 180 / 2.2 = 82 | 82 kg x 0.8 = 66 g |
| 210 | 210 / 2.2 = 95 | 95 kg x 0.8 = 76 g |

There is some debate among researchers as to whether the amino acid histidine should be classified as essential or nonessential, sometimes also referred to as indispensable or dispensable, respectively. The WHO 2007 report states: "To date, the indispensability of histidine in healthy adults remains unresolved." So that nothing potentially important is missed, histidine is included in the analyses of essential amino acid requirements in various foods and raw food diets examined throughout this chapter and elsewhere in the book.

Also note that two of the essential amino acids, methionine and phenylalanine, are both paired up with a nonessential amino acid. Methionine is paired with cysteine, while phenylalanine is paired with tyrosine. Methionine can be converted into cysteine by the body, and this conversion takes place as needed. If there's an ample supply of cysteine from food, the body doesn't have to rely as much on conversion from methionine. That's why the WHO looks at methionine and cysteine combined in order to give its best recommendation. The relationship between phenylalanine and tyrosine works the same way as the relationship between methionine and cysteine. In all of the figures throughout this chapter, the sum total of methionine and cysteine is listed simply as methionine, and the sum total of phenylalanine and tyrosine is listed simply as phenylalanine.

**Table 4.2.** Recommended essential amino acid intake

| Essential amino acid | WHO recommendations (mg/kg) | Recommended intake (g) for individual weighing 150 lbs (68 kg) |
|---|---|---|
| Histidine | 10 | 0.68 |
| Isoleucine | 20 | 1.36 |
| Leucine | 39 | 2.65 |
| Lysine | 30 | 2.04 |
| Methionine (+ cysteine) | 15 total | 1.02 total |
| Phenylalanine (+ tyrosine) | 25 total | 1.70 total |
| Threonine | 15 | 1.02 |
| Tryptophan | 4 | 0.27 |
| Valine | 26 | 1.77 |

For a 150-pound (68 kg) person, if any particular food or combination of foods can supply 54 grams of total protein (see table 4.1), including the specified quantity of each of the essential amino acids (see table 4.2, page 31, and figure 4.1 on the facing page), then all the protein recommendations for this individual have been met. When an adequate amount of calories from food supplies all the total protein and all the essential amino acids in sufficient quantities for an individual's needs, the protein in that food is known as complete protein. If either total protein or at least one essential amino acid is supplied in insufficient quantities, the protein source(s) in question are said to supply incomplete protein.

In the following figures, we'll examine the total protein and essential amino acid content of 2,500 calories from individual foods and sample raw food diets. This number of calories is the suggested intake for a 5-foot, 10-inch, 150-pound (68 kg), 40-year-old male who is moderately active, using the Harris-Benedict equation, a formula that provides an estimate of calorie needs based on height, weight, age, sex, and activity level. (See Computing Calorie needs on pages 126–128 for more details.) The equation suggests 1,946 calories if this person were sedentary.

If your height, weight, age, sex, or activity level is different from our model person, you can use the Harris-Benedict equation to estimate your individual calorie needs. You can then compare the protein and essential amino acid levels in various foods and diets at that calorie level to your individual total protein and essential amino acid recommendations, much like we will be doing in this chapter with our model person. If you're larger or smaller, both your calorie and protein needs will go up or down together proportionally.

I'm not suggesting you derive all your calories each day from only one food, but an appropriate amount must be chosen to see if a daily caloric intake of those foods can supply the amount of total protein and essential amino acids recommended by the WHO. Any food, no matter how high in protein, cannot supply an individual with all their total protein and essential amino acid requirements if an inadequate amount of calories from that food is consumed. Chicken eggs, for example, are touted to be high in complete protein. If someone consumed only 400 calories per day of chicken eggs, the protein from those 400 calories would be incomplete when daily needs are considered. This fact alone doesn't make eggs an inadequate food. It simply means a more reasonable amount of calories must be consumed to supply appropriate quantities of key nutrients, such as total protein and essential amino acids.

In addition, comparing the same number of calories from different foods is necessary to create a fair comparison between the foods examined.

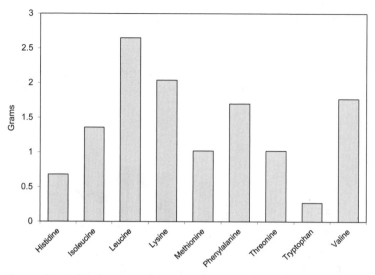

**Figure 4.1.** WHO daily essential amino acid recommendations for a 150-pound person

## Amino Acids in Various Foods

We're now ready to examine the total protein and essential amino acid content of different foods and different diets. We'll compare this content with the recommendations established by the 2007 WHO report for our model person. There are many other foods we could have added to each category to analyze, but the examples used in this chapter provide an accurate assessment of the protein content of different foods and different raw food diets.

### Vegetables

Initially, I'll show the total protein content of 2,500 calories' worth of various vegetables. Again, I'm by no means suggesting that someone get all their calories each day from only one food, but this serves as a useful illustration of the total protein and essential amino acid quantities in a day's worth of calories.

Figure 4.2 on the next page shows that a day's worth of calories obtained from any of the vegetables listed (or any combination thereof) meets the recommended total protein intake. Most of these vegetables actually exceed the total protein recommendations by a very substantial margin. However, it would be nearly impossible to obtain a full day's worth of calories from many of these vegetables, which would require more chewing, time, patience, and digestive space than most people have. But with such a high amount of protein per calorie, even a relatively small number of calories of many of these vegetables can add a significant amount of protein. Eating vegetables is also a great way to get a lot of fiber, vitamins, minerals, phytonutrients, antioxidants, and essential fats.

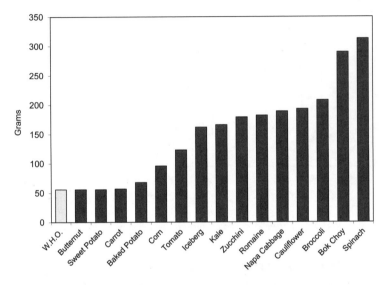

**Figure 4.2.** Total protein content of 2,500 calories of various vegetables versus WHO recommendations for a 150-pound person

Figures 4.3 through 4.10 on pages 35–38 show each of the vegetables charted in figure 4.2 and compare their essential amino acid content against the WHO recommendations. Figure 4.2 shows that 2,500 calories' worth of these vegetables does a great job of supplying a day's total protein for someone of this weight, and figures 4.3 through 4.10 show that each of these vegetables also supply more than ample quantities of each essential amino acid. Corn, while botanically a grain, is listed in this section as it is used as a vegetable from both a culinary and commonly understood point of view. It's listed by itself to give special emphasis to the fact that an adequate amount of calories from corn can create a complete protein. We'll consider the essential amino acid profile of corn, along with wheat, later in this chapter.

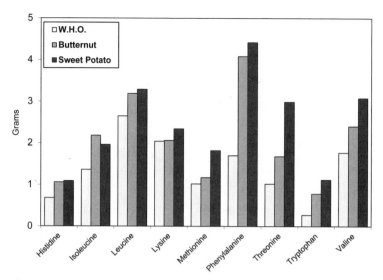

**Figure 4.3.** Essential amino acid content of 2,500 calories of butternut squash and sweet potato versus WHO recommendations for a 150-pound person

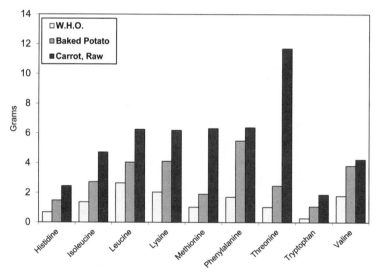

**Figure 4.4.** Essential amino acid content of 2,500 calories of baked potato and carrot versus WHO recommendations for a 150-pound person

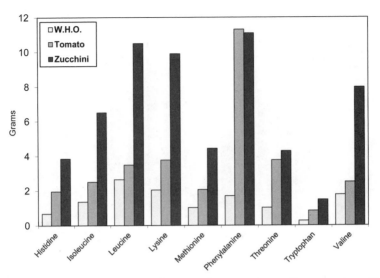

**Figure 4.5.** Essential amino acid content of 2,500 calories of tomato and zucchini versus WHO recommendations for a 150-pound person

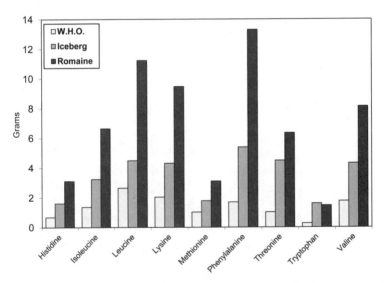

**Figure 4.6.** Essential amino acid content of 2,500 calories of iceberg lettuce and romaine lettuce versus WHO recommendations for a 150-pound person

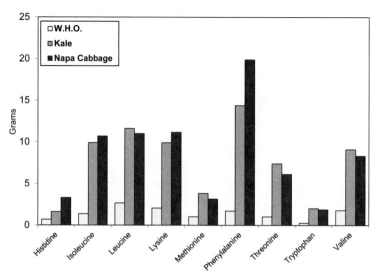

**Figure 4.7.** Essential amino acid content of 2,500 calories of kale and napa cabbage versus WHO recommendations for a 150-pound person

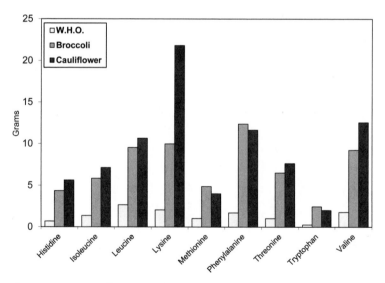

**Figure 4.8.** Essential amino acid content of 2,500 calories of broccoli and cauliflower versus WHO recommendations for a 150-pound person

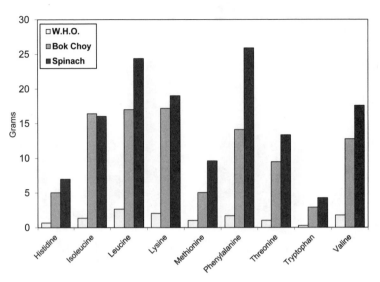

**Figure 4.9.** Essential amino acid content of 2,500 calories of bok choy and spinach versus WHO recommendations for a 150-pound person

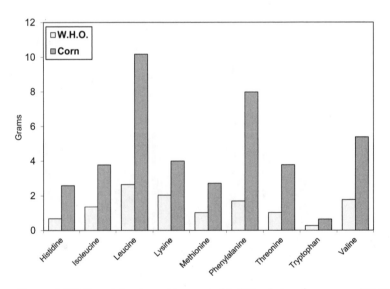

**Figure 4.10.** Essential amino acid content of 2,500 calories of corn versus WHO recommendations for a 150-pound person

## Nuts and Seeds

Similar analyses on a sampling of nuts and seeds in figures 4.11 through 4.15 on pages 39–41 show a plant food that's an incomplete protein: macadamia nuts. Not only are they deficient in total protein, they're also lacking in several essential amino acids. Considering the amounts of the amino acids isoleucine, leucine, tryptophan, and even valine, one could potentially argue that macadamia nuts provide pretty close to the conservative overestimates recommended by the WHO and are therefore probably adequate for most people. The levels of lysine and methionine, however, are not even close. Because macadamia nuts provide 94 percent of their calories from fat, there's little room left for protein. The remaining nuts and seeds easily supply more than enough total protein and all the essential amino acids in a sample day's worth of calories.

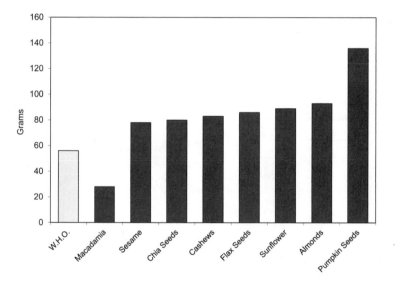

**Figure 4.11.** Total protein content of 2,500 calories of various nuts or seeds versus WHO recommendations for a 150-pound person

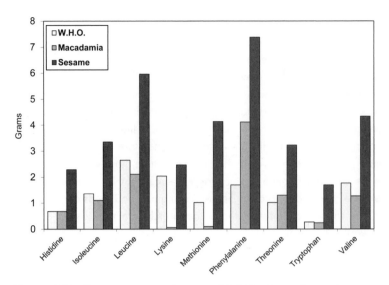

**Figure 4.12.** Essential amino acid content of 2,500 calories of macadamia nuts and sesame seeds versus WHO recommendations for a 150-pound person

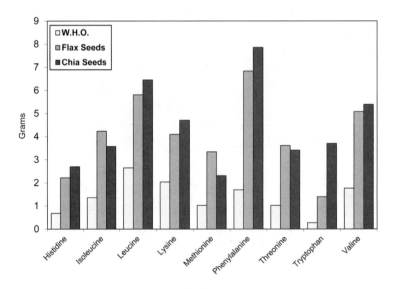

**Figure 4.13.** Essential amino acid content of 2,500 calories of flaxseeds and chia seeds versus WHO recommendations for a 150-pound person

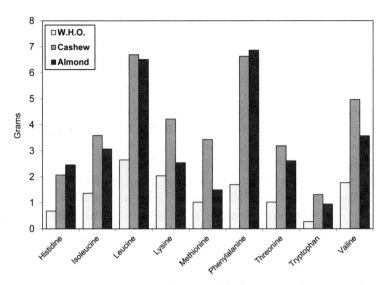

**Figure 4.14.** Essential amino acid content of 2,500 calories of cashews and almonds versus WHO recommendations for a 150-pound person

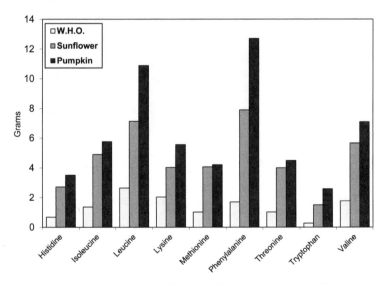

**Figure 4.15.** Essential amino acid content of 2,500 calories of sunflower and pumpkin seeds versus WHO recommendations for a 150-pound person

## Fruits

A sampling of commonly consumed fruits in figures 4.16 through 4.19 on pages 42–44 shows that fruit alone does not do the best job of meeting WHO total protein and essential amino acid recommendations, which are conservatively overestimated.

Because other foods, such as vegetables, need to be included in a healthy diet to provide a well-rounded nutrient profile, I'm not concerned about fruit alone not meeting all of the WHO protein recommendations, any more than I am concerned that vegetables alone will not meet all of the calorie needs for an individual. In other words, foods other than fruit need to be included in a sustainably healthy diet and can also increase the protein content to more than recommended levels, as we will see shortly.

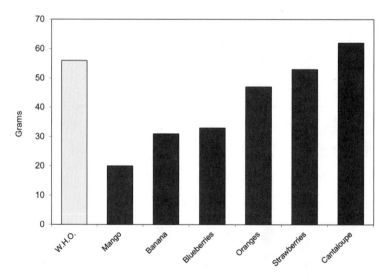

**Figure 4.16.** Total protein content of 2,500 calories of each fruit versus WHO recommendations for a 150-pound person

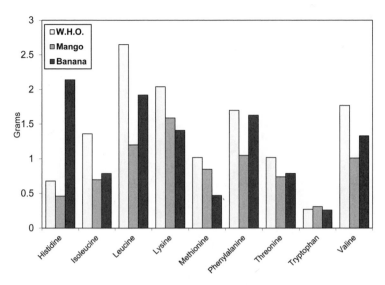

**Figure 4.17.** Essential amino acid content of 2,500 calories of mango and banana versus WHO recommendations for a 150-pound person

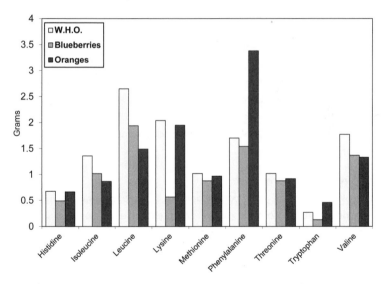

**Figure 4.18.** Essential amino acid content of 2,500 calories of blueberries and oranges versus WHO recommendations for a 150-pound person

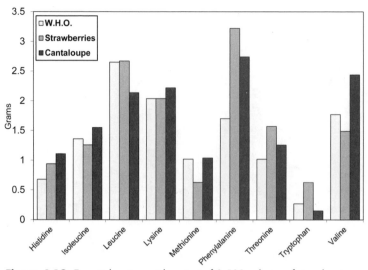

**Figure 4.19.** Essential amino acid content of 2,500 calories of strawberries and cantaloupe versus WHO recommendations for a 150-pound person

## Protein and Amino Acids in Sample Raw Food Diets

As the majority of calories on a raw food diet typically come from the foods we just examined, fruits, vegetables, and nuts and seeds, we'll analyze three sample raw food diets composed of different proportions of these staple raw foods before we go on to analyze the total protein and essential amino acid content of other plant foods. This will allow us to see how well actual raw diets compare to WHO recommendations for total protein and essential amino acids. The following graphs are provided to analyze three typical raw diets: high-sweet fruit, low-sweet fruit, and intermediate raw (moderate fruit-moderate fat).

### High-Sweet Fruit Raw Diet

The sample diet on the next page contains a large quantity of food but only provides 2,051 calories. It's a great example of how eating predominantly fruits and vegetables within a reasonable range of calories can easily provide adequate protein. For our model person, who should consume 2,500 calories a day according to the Harris-Benedict equation, this lower-calorie diet would supply the total recommended protein and exceed the required level of each essential amino acid, as shown in figures 4.20 and 4.21 on page 46. In contrast, a total fruit diet of either 2,051 or 2,500 calories would usually not meet the total protein and essential amino acid recommendations. There were enough vegetables in our sample diet to meet and exceed all the recommendations. Leafy greens

**Breakfast**
1 large cantaloupe (1,360 g)

**Lunch**
4 medium bananas (472 g)
5 cups (227 g) chopped romaine lettuce
1½ cups (227 g) fresh blueberries

**Afternoon Snack**
13 fresh apricots (454 g)
5 fresh figs (250 g)

**Dinner**
Soup
3¾ cups (340 g) chopped broccoli
2 medium bell peppers, chopped (227 g)
1¼ cups (227 g) chopped tomatoes
5 leaves fresh basil (2.5 g)

Salad
5 cups (227 g) chopped romaine lettuce
2¼ cups (227 g) diced celery
½ to ⅔ bunch baby spinach (227 g)

Salad Dressing
Mango, pit and skin removed (207 g)
Juice of 1 lemon (3 oz/84 g)
1 tablespoon (15 g) sesame tahini

and many other vegetables are so high in protein that including reasonable quantities of them, along with a substantial quantity of fruit, can easily meet protein recommendations, even considering the recommendations are based on conservative overestimates and the sample diet has a significant calorie deficit for our moderately active model person.

If the quantities of food in this high-sweet fruit diet were increased in order to provide 2,500 calories, the total protein and essential amino acid profiles would be as shown in figures 4.22 and 4.23 on page 47. The total protein and essential amino acid levels exceed every recommendation by an even greater margin than 2,051 calories of the same foods. Even at a calorie deficit for a sedentary person, there is still enough protein for most people.

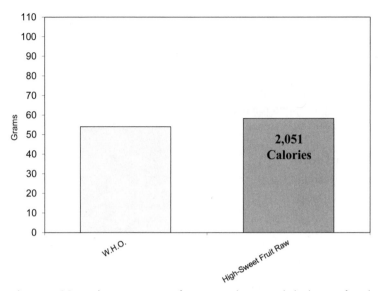

**Figure 4.20.** Total protein content of a 2,051-calorie sample high-sweet fruit diet versus WHO recommendation

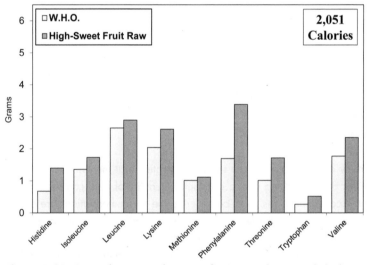

**Figure 4.21.** Essential amino acid content of a 2,051-calorie sample high-sweet fruit diet versus WHO recommendations for a 150-pound person

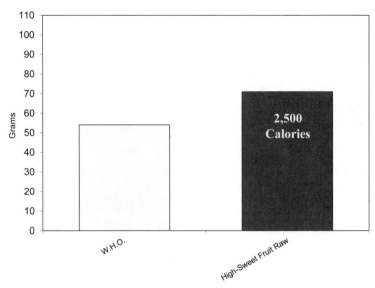

**Figure 4.22.** Total protein content of a 2,500-calorie sample high-sweet fruit diet versus WHO recommendation

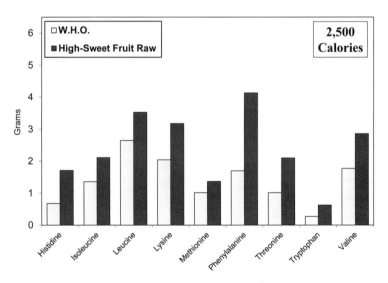

**Figure 4.23.** Essential amino acid content of a 2,500-calorie sample high-sweet fruit diet versus WHO recommendations for a 150-pound person

### Low-Sweet Fruit Raw Diet

The menu on the next page also has a substantial quantity of food (although not as much as the one on page 45), but the entire menu supplies just over 2,000 calories. Even though that's nearly 500 calories less than our moderately active model person would need, figures 4.24 and 4.25 show that this menu would still supply more than enough total protein and all the essential amino acids. As nuts and seeds are higher in protein than fruit, this menu has a bit more protein than the previous one. If the amount of food was increased to bring it up to 2,500 calories, as shown in figures 4.26 and 4.27 on page 50, all the recommendations would be exceeded by an even larger margin. Even at a calorie deficit for a sedentary person, there is still plenty of protein.

## Breakfast

Blended Quinoa Cereal
½ cup (85 g) dry quinoa, sprouted (approximate yield: 1 cup)
½ cup (237 ml) water
½ ripe banana (59 g)
½ teaspoon (1.3 g) cinnamon
½ cup (71.5 g) unsoaked almonds, for garnish (if soaked, approximate yield: 1 cup)

## Lunch

Sprouted Lentil and Vegetable Soup
2 cups (202 g) chopped celery
1 cup (180 g) chopped tomatoes
⅓ cup (64 g) dry lentils, sprouted (approximate yield: 1⅓ cups)
½ medium avocado (68 g)
1 green onion (25 g)

## Dinner

Salad
4 cups (188 g) chopped romaine lettuce
4 cups (99 g) chopped dandelion greens
1 cup (180 g) chopped tomatoes
1 cup (110 g) grated carrots
1 cup (104 g) chopped cucumber
½ cup (21.2 g) chopped fresh basil

Salad Dressing
2 cups (298 g) chopped red bell pepper
2 cups (248 g) chopped zucchini
½ cup (122 g) fresh-squeezed lemon juice
2 tablespoons (18 g) almonds
2 tablespoons (20 g) chia seeds
2 tablespoons (18 g) unhulled sesame seeds

## Evening Snack

¼ cup (36 g) almonds

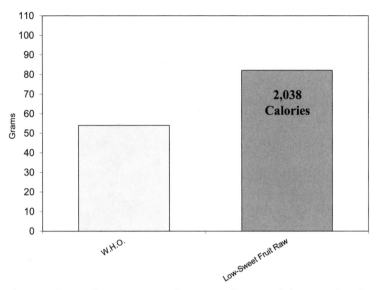

**Figure 4.24.** Total protein content of a 2,038-calorie sample low-sweet fruit diet versus WHO recommendation

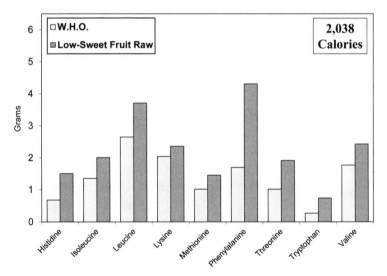

**Figure 4.25.** Essential amino acid content of a 2,038-calorie sample low-sweet fruit diet versus WHO recommendations for a 150-pound person

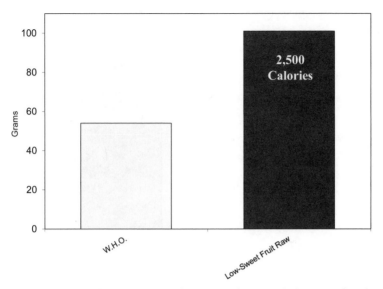

**Figure 4.26.** Total protein content of a 2,500-calorie sample low-sweet fruit diet versus WHO recommendation

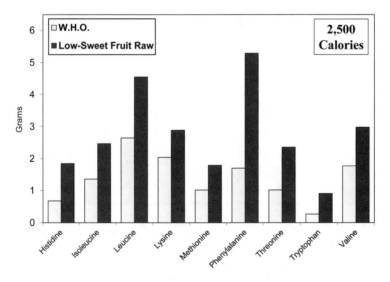

**Figure 4.27.** Essential amino acid content of a 2,500-calorie sample low-sweet fruit diet versus WHO recommendations for a 150-pound person

### Intermediate Raw Diet (Moderate Fruit-Moderate Fat)

The following sample intermediate raw diet below consists of a mixture of fruits, vegetables, nuts, and seeds. Once again, this large quantity of food doesn't provide an excess of calories for our model person. Figures 4.28 and 4.29 on the next page show that a 2,000-calorie diet will exceed the total protein and essential amino acids needed to meet the recommendations for our model person by a substantial margin. When the amount of food is increased to 2,500 calories, as shown in figures 4.30 and 4.31 on page 53, the recommendations are exceeded by an even greater margin. Even at a calorie deficit for a sedentary person, there is once again plenty of protein.

### Breakfast
1 medium (814 g) cantaloupe

### Lunch
Green Smoothie
4 cups (268 g) chopped kale
2¾ cups (425 g) chopped mangoes
1 cup (237 ml) fresh-squeezed orange juice
2 medium (236 g) bananas

### Dinner
Salad
5 cups (227 g) chopped romaine lettuce
3½ cups (400 g) shredded zucchini
1 head (700 g) cauliflower
2 (364 g) red tomatoes

Salad Dressing
2 medium (392 g) zucchini
¼ cup (61 g) fresh-squeezed lemon juice
¼ cup (36 g) unhulled sesame seeds, soaked
¼ cup (36 g) almonds, soaked
1 tablespoon (10.3 g) flaxseeds

### Snack
Handful of almonds (35 g)

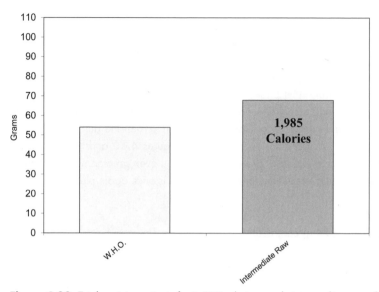

**Figure 4.28.** Total protein content of a 1,985-calorie sample intermediate raw diet versus WHO recommendation

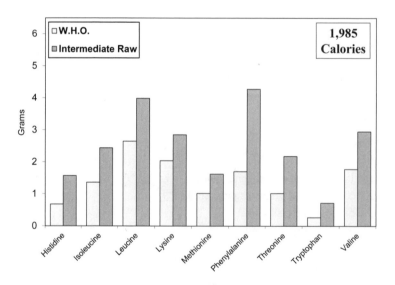

**Figure 4.29.** Essential amino acid content of a 1,985-calorie sample intermediate raw diet versus WHO recommendations for a 150-pound person

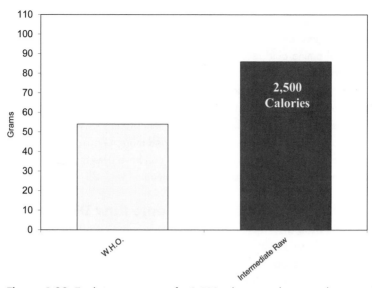

**Figure 4.30.** Total protein content of a 2,500-calorie sample intermediate raw diet versus WHO recommendation

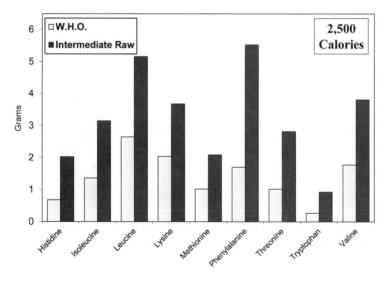

**Figure 4.31.** Essential amino acid content of a 2,500-calorie sample intermediate raw diet versus WHO recommendations for a 150-pound person

In all three of these examples, a raw food diet consisting of different proportions of vegetables, fruit, nuts, and seeds easily supplied all the total protein and essential amino acid recommendations, even when the total calorie content was around 500 calories below recommendations for our model person's height, weight, sex, age, and activity level. This can help people feel confident that they are getting what they need, even when weight loss is desired. In addition, as these raw plant foods have such excellent profiles for vitamins, minerals, antioxidants, phytonutrients, fiber, water, and more, people who choose a diet based on whole, natural, raw plant foods can have even more confidence in the healthfulness of this approach to good nutrition.

## Additional Foods Included in Some Raw Diets
### Sea Vegetables and Spirulina
Some raw-food enthusiasts include sea vegetables in their diets, while others do not. Those who do, however, usually don't consume a significant percentage of their daily calories from them. Nevertheless, it seemed fitting to include the same protein analysis that we've done with the raw food staples thus far. There are not many analyses of sea vegetables available in the USDA nutrient database, but with the handful shown in figures 4.32 through 4.34, it's apparent that total protein and all the essential amino acids are supplied in great abundance. This is true to an extreme degree with spirulina.

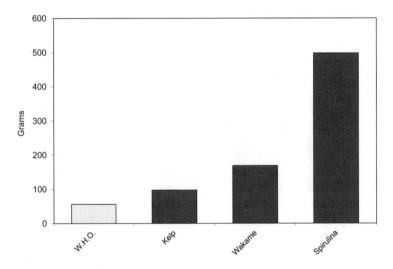

**Figure 4.32.** Total protein content of 2,500 calories of each sea vegetable versus WHO recommendations for a 150-pound person

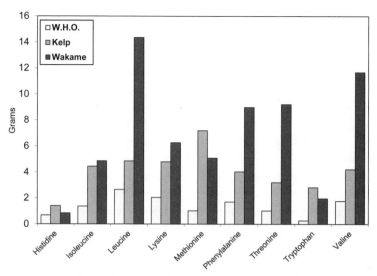

**Figure 4.33.** Essential amino acid content of 2,500 calories of kelp and wakame versus WHO recommendations for a 150-pound person

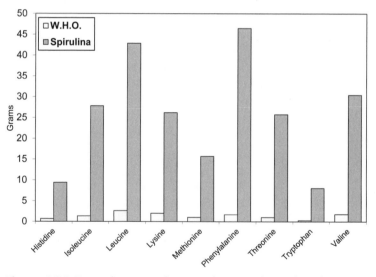

**Figure 4.34.** Essential amino acid content of 2,500 calories of spirulina versus WHO recommendations for a 150-pound person

## Grains

This book is primarily about raw food diets, and not many raw-food enthusiasts consume an abundance of grains. Some do, however, usually in sprouted form. And not all people who base their diets on raw foods eat exclusively raw. Some of the cooked foods consumed are whole grains and pseudograins, such as brown rice, oats, and quinoa. Therefore, I felt it was worth examining the amino acid content of grains to identify sources of protein in a plant-based diet, especially considering that most people believe grains as a group of foods provide incomplete protein.

For total protein, 2,500 calories of brown rice meets the WHO recommendations for 97.5 percent of the population. All the other grains listed in figure 4.35 exceed the recommendations. However, despite exceeding the total protein content, a full day's worth of calories from millet has only about 75 percent of the recommended amount of lysine, as shown in figure 4.36. Even though those recommendations are based on conservative overestimates, there's no good reason to take a chance on getting less of an essential amino acid than needed, especially when it's so easy to get enough. There are many other foods, including other grains, that contain far more lysine than millet.

Many nutritionists have stated that grains in general are insufficient in lysine, and while this appears to be true for a few of them, such a blanket statement is not supported by the facts, as indicated in figures 4.36 through 4.41 (pages 57-59). Lysine is supplied in the least abundance compared to the other essential amino acids, in general. Also note that although they are not true grains botanically, amaranth, quinoa, and buckwheat are included in this section as they are used as grains from both a culinary and commonly understood point of view. For more information on this, see pages 7-8. The essential amino acid content of wheat is analyzed again along with corn on page 67.

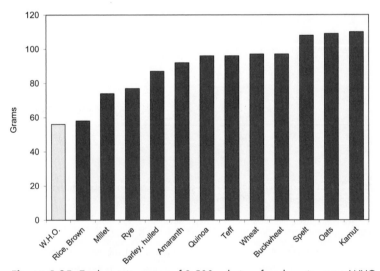

**Figure 4.35.** Total protein content of 2,500 calories of each grain versus WHO recommendations for a 150-pound person

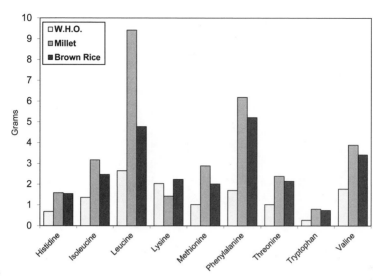

**Figure 4.36.** Essential amino acid content of 2,500 calories of millet and brown rice versus WHO recommendations for a 150-pound person

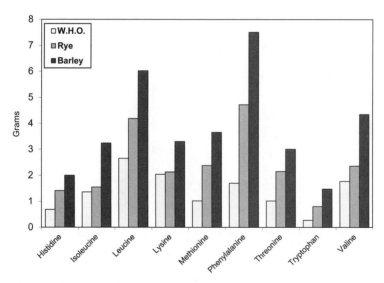

**Figure 4.37.** Essential amino acid content of 2,500 calories of rye and barley versus WHO recommendations for a 150-pound person

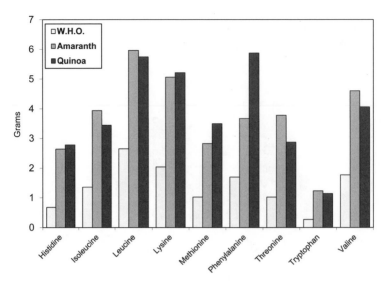

**Figure 4.38.** Essential amino acid content of 2,500 calories of amaranth and quinoa versus WHO recommendations for a 150-pound person

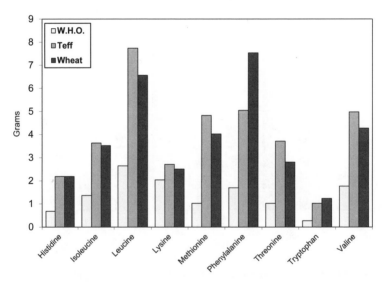

**Figure 4.39.** Essential amino acid content of 2,500 calories of teff and wheat versus WHO recommendations for a 150-pound person

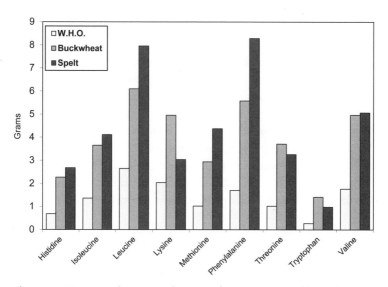

**Figure 4.40.** Essential amino acid content of 2,500 calories of buckwheat and spelt versus WHO recommendations for a 150-pound person

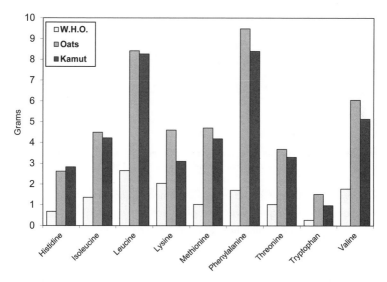

**Figure 4.41.** Essential amino acid content of 2,500 calories of oats and Kamut versus WHO recommendations for a 150-pound person

So far, these samples have only included whole grains, but most of the grains consumed in typical modern diets are refined grains. As it turns out, refined grains have considerably less total protein and essential amino acid content than their unrefined counterparts. Twenty-five hundred calories of whole wheat flour has 97 grams of total protein, whereas the same number of calories of refined wheat flour has 71 grams of total protein. The same calculations for brown versus white rice are 58 grams and 52 grams, respectively, and hulled (whole grain) barley and pearl (refined) barley have 88 grams and 46 grams of total protein, respectively. Figures 4.42 through 4.44 show the essential amino acid content of the same amount of calories of these three whole-grain products compared to the refined-grain products.

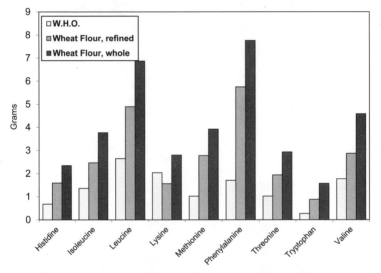

**Figure 4.42.** Essential amino acid content of 2,500 calories of refined wheat flour and whole wheat flour versus WHO recommendations for a 150-pound person

Clearly, the total protein and essential amino acid content of each whole grain is considerably higher than that of its refined counterpart. The only exception is brown rice, which has a slightly lower methionine content than white rice. Figures 4.39 and 4.42 show that wheat flour and whole wheat flour both exceed the lysine recommendations by a notable margin. Figure 4.42 shows that the lysine content of refined wheat flour is only about half that of whole wheat flour, illustrating that if someone consumed a full day's worth of calories from refined wheat flour, they would clearly get less than the recommended amount of lysine. Figures 4.43 and 4.44 show similar scenarios for whole versus refined rice and barley.

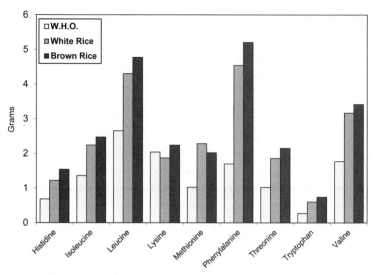

**Figure 4.43.** Essential amino acid content of 2,500 calories of white rice and brown rice versus WHO recommendations for a 150-pound person

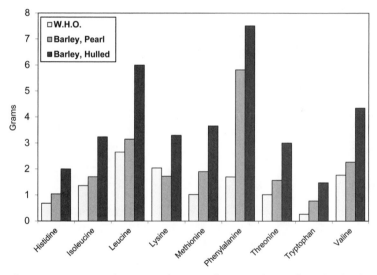

**Figure 4.44.** Essential amino acid content of 2,500 calories of pearl (refined) barley and hulled barley (only the outer hull taken off to reveal the whole grain) versus WHO recommendations for a 150-pound person

I don't support the consumption of refined grains, so their lower protein content is not a major concern. They're lacking in fiber, higher on the glycemic index, more calorie dense, and are missing many of the important nutrients found in their unrefined counterparts. In addition, refined grains usually come packaged with a host of undesirable ingredients, such as hydrogenated omega-6 (pro-inflammatory) oils, refined sweeteners, and preservatives. If you prefer not to consume grains at all, there are many other foods to choose from that supply plenty of protein, such as fruits, vegetables, nuts, and seeds.

## Beans

This book is primarily about raw food diets, and not many raw-food enthusiasts consume an abundance of beans. Some do, however, usually in sprouted form, and not all people who base their diets on raw foods eat exclusively raw. Therefore I felt it was worth examining the amino acid content of beans as we identify sources of protein in a plant-based diet. Examples of popular sprouted legumes are lentils, mung beans, and peas. Note that some legumes in their raw or sprouted form, such as kidney beans, are not recommended and should not be consumed because of the presence of problematic substances, such as phytohemagglutinin, which can lead to gastrointestinal illness. I would encourage you to research legumes to find out which are suitable for sprouting.

An analysis of ten different types of beans is shown in figures 4.45 through 4.50 on pages 62–65, first for total protein and then for essential amino acid content. These figures display similar results as those found with vegetables. Every one of the beans analyzed supplies an abundance of both total protein and each essential amino acid, making them complete proteins.

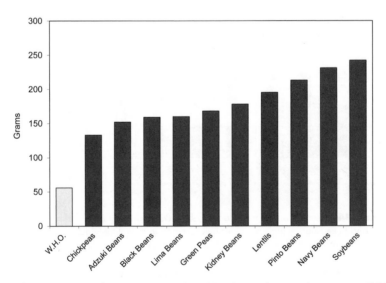

**Figure 4.45.** Total protein content of 2,500 calories of various beans versus WHO recommendations for a 150-pound person

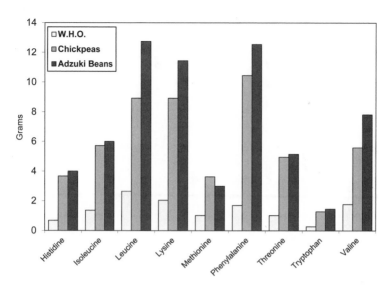

**Figure 4.46.** Essential amino acid content of 2,500 calories of chickpeas and adzuki beans versus WHO recommendations for a 150-pound person

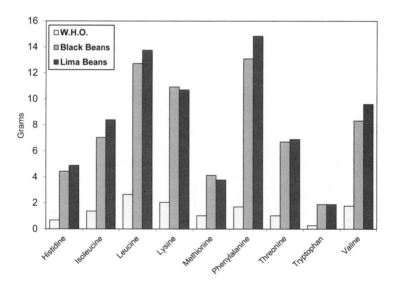

**Figure 4.47.** Essential amino acid content of 2,500 calories of black beans and lima beans versus WHO recommendations for a 150-pound person

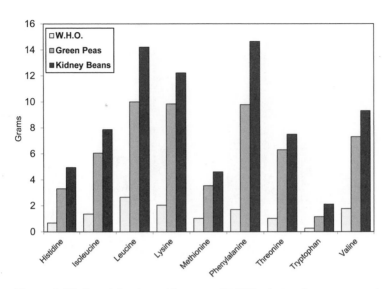

**Figure 4.48.** Essential amino acid content of 2,500 calories of green peas and kidney beans versus WHO recommendations for a 150-pound person

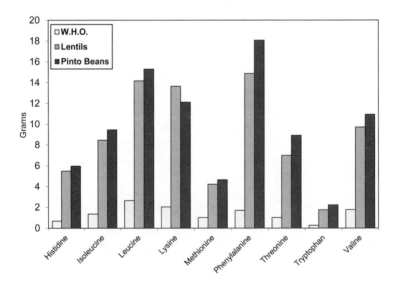

**Figure 4.49.** Essential amino acid content of 2,500 calories of lentils and pinto beans versus WHO recommendations for a 150-pound person

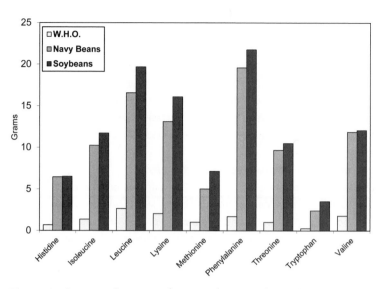

**Figure 4.50.** Essential amino acid content of 2,500 calories of navy beans and soybeans versus WHO recommendations for a 150-pound person

## Protein Deficiency on a Raw Food Diet

There are a few ways in which a raw food diet might not supply enough total protein or one or more of the essential amino acids. If there aren't enough total calories consumed (for example, if someone ate only 400 calories a day over a period of time), it's likely the diet would be lacking in protein. This could happen on any diet, not just a raw food diet, as was shown on page 32 with eggs.

Another way someone eating a raw diet could be lacking in protein is if they rely too much on processed foods that contain no protein, such as any type of oil or most refined sweeteners. Oil is extremely calorie dense, so small amounts can supply a lot of calories, but no protein at all. Most concentrated sweeteners can also add a lot of calories but no protein. Even though these ingredients may be raw or allegedly raw, they are not necessarily health promoting. One of the major reasons for eating raw foods is to experience the health benefits from consuming them, and eating processed and refined foods is in direct opposition to this goal.

Raw diets based exclusively on fruit may not meet all the WHO recommendations. However, fruit-based diets can easily supply complete protein as long as meaningful quantities of vegetables, such as those shown in the high-sweet fruit and intermediate raw diets on pages 130 and 137, are included as well.

The bottom line is that any rationally implemented diet based on varying amounts of fresh fruit, meaningful quantities of vegetables, and various amounts of optional nuts and seeds and other foods—that supplies sufficient calorie intake (even when reasonable weight loss is desired)—can provide more than adequate amounts of total protein and each essential amino acid. A raw food diet lacking in protein or any one or more of the essential amino acids would have to be extreme and unhealthful. The resulting protein deficiency would then have to do with inappropriate choices, as opposed to any lack from the whole plant foods consumed on a rationally implemented raw food diet.

### Wheat and Corn Compared to Human Milk

In studies conducted in the United States by longtime collaborators Thomas Osborne and Lafayette Mendel from 1911 to 1914, wheat and corn were deemed partially incomplete and incomplete protein sources, respectively. This was because young laboratory rats did not grow and develop properly when their only source of protein was wheat or corn. Wheat was found to be low in the essential amino acid lysine, while corn was found to be low in lysine and tryptophan, at least for growing rats. In contrast, protein from cow's milk resulted in normal growth and development for rats and was therefore deemed a complete protein. This was groundbreaking research at the time, as protein quality studies had never been conducted with living organisms before. These conclusions were then extrapolated to estimate human requirements, which created a lot of confusion.

It wasn't until the 1940s that Dr. William Rose of the University of Illinois determined the total protein and essential amino acid requirements for human beings. Dr. Rose had previously built upon Osborne and Mendel's research to determine total protein and essential amino acid requirements in rats, which laid the groundwork needed to conduct human trials. He found that the total protein and essential amino acid requirements of rats and humans differed significantly. Rats have higher overall protein and essential amino acid requirements than human beings do and need at least one more essential amino acid. Rat's milk, for example, supplies 26 percent of its calories from protein, while human milk supplies 5.5 percent of its calories from protein. While 5.5 percent of the calories from protein may sound low, human milk supplies all the total protein and each of the essential amino acids in sufficient quantities for the normal growth and development of a human newborn.

In an admittedly unusual yet useful analysis, figures 4.51 and 4.52 show the total protein and essential amino acid profiles of 2,500 calories from human milk compared to the same amount of calories of wheat and corn. Calorie per calorie, wheat and corn supply far greater amounts of total protein and almost all the essential amino acids when compared to human milk. Lysine in wheat and tryptophan in corn are the exceptions, as they are supplied in quantities roughly equal to human milk. Given this direct comparison, it would only make sense that if human milk is considered a complete protein, wheat and corn would be as well.

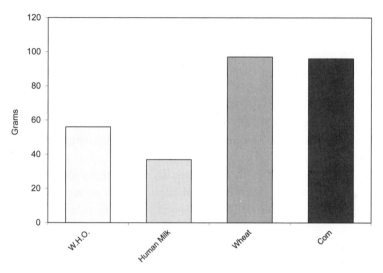

**Figure 4.51.** Total protein content of 2,500 calories of human milk, wheat, and corn versus WHO recommendations for a 150-pound person

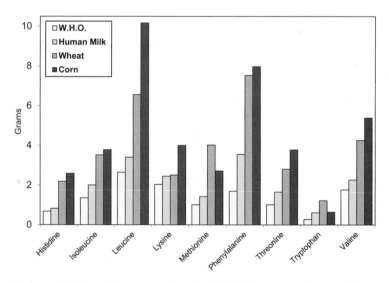

**Figure 4.52.** Essential amino acid content of 2,500 calories of human milk, wheat, and corn versus WHO recommendations for a 150-pound person

Conversely, if people consider wheat and corn to be incomplete proteins, it would follow that human milk would also be an incomplete protein. That doesn't make any sense in reality, as babies have been consuming mothers' milk often as their only source of protein since the beginning of human history and have grown and developed properly as a result.

Please understand, this is for illustration purposes only! I'm not suggesting that an adult consume any quantity of milk from a human or any other mammal, given that milk is intended for developing infants of the same species. This analysis is simply an exercise to show that we may wish to reconsider how we think about complete and incomplete proteins, and if research on one species can always be accurately extrapolated to another.

We're often told that most plant proteins are incomplete and that only a select few are complete, such as soy or quinoa. As it turns out, it's the other way around. Most of the whole plant foods we analyzed provide complete protein when the recommended amount of calories for our moderately active model person was consumed. Our sampling of vegetables, nuts, seeds, sea vegetables, whole grains, and beans show that most plant proteins are complete proteins, while only a few are incomplete. It would be an exception to have incomplete protein from plants, rather than the rule.

### The Effects of Heat on Protein Bioavailability

We've all seen how heat can affect both the texture and flavor of foods. When batter turns into pancakes or muffins, bread becomes toast, or meat is grilled or roasted, various chemical reactions occur that wouldn't have happened if it weren't for the presence of heat. Some substances are lost, some are transformed, and new substances are formed.

A classic example of heat changing the structure of protein in food is that of egg whites, which change from clear and runny when raw to white and solid once cooked. Egg whites are composed predominantly of protein, so the fact that the taste and texture of egg whites change when subjected to heat indicates that the protein structure they're made from changes as a result of exposure to heat.

Each amino acid has its own unique structure, and that makes some amino acids more susceptible to the effects of heat than others, with lysine being the most susceptible. As the structure of lysine and other substances in a food change during the cooking process, this new form of lysine can now react with certain other newly formed substances to form new products, which were not present in the food before it was heated. Because it's now part of a new product, the lysine is no longer biologically available to be utilized as an individual amino acid. Lysine in this form is known as blocked lysine, or inactivated lysine. A study done at the University of Kiel in Germany found that well over 50 percent of the lysine in foods may become blocked, depending upon the food and the heating method, with higher heat and longer cooking times causing greater lysine blockage. Other essential amino acids known to be similarly altered as a result of exposure to heat include tryptophan, methionine, threonine, leucine, and isoleucine.

When we heat and process foods, we significantly decrease the biological availability of the proteins in those foods. Raw, unheated foods therefore supply protein of greater biological availability than their cooked and processed counterparts.

It's interesting to note that most diets are composed primarily of foods that have been cooked or processed in a way that renders many of the amino acids they contain biologically unavailable. Despite this, the modern human population is not suffering from widespread protein deficiency in the presence of adequate caloric intake. We've seen very clearly that raw food diets based on varying proportions of fruits, vegetables, and nuts and seeds can easily supply all the total protein and essential amino acids in more than sufficient quantities to meet the conservatively overestimated human protein recommendations. When we consider that the protein in raw foods has not been compromised by heat, there should be even less of a concern regarding the adequacy of protein in raw food diets.

## CHAPTER 5

# Minerals

---

MINERALS, OR ELEMENTS, FORM THE BASIC CONSTITUENTS OF MATTER. Like vitamins and fiber, minerals play important and diverse roles in the body. They don't provide calories but are important for numerous functions, such as the conversion of carbohydrate, protein, and fat into energy. Minerals are primarily derived from the earth, with over 100 individual minerals identified so far. Some of these are essential for human health, and the principle way that they're obtained is through the diet. The information that follows includes some of the most important minerals for human health, their functions in the body, and good raw food sources.

The US Institute of Medicine (IOM) has given recommendations for the minimum amount of minerals, vitamins, and other nutrients it feels are necessary for health. Like the WHO, which has set recommendations for protein intake, the IOM has set Recommended Dietary Allowances (RDAs) when the amount of a nutrient need is well documented. The IOM also recommends adequate intakes (AIs) when the needed amount is not as well documented. Throughout this chapter and the chapter on vitamins, these nutrient levels will be provided, if known. In addition, the IOM reports upper limits (ULs) for nutrients when there's a known toxicity level. Combined, these levels are called Dietary Reference Intakes (DRIs).

## Calcium

Calcium is the most abundant mineral in the human body, with 99 percent found in the bones and teeth and 1 percent found in blood and tissues. It's important to consume enough dietary calcium, and the adequate intake (AI) of calcium for adults is 1,000 milligrams per day for women up to and including 50 years and men up to and including 70 years. The AI for women 51 and over and men over 70 is 1,200 milligrams per day.

### Sources of Calcium

The cabbage and sunflower plant families contain some of the richest sources of calcium in the plant kingdom. Kale is often prized for its rich mineral content, especially calcium. Bok choy, napa cabbage, mustard greens, and other members of the cabbage family are also notable sources of this important mineral. Per calorie, watercress contains one of the highest amounts of calcium in this family. Dandelion greens, a member of the sunflower family, are very calcium-rich, as are romaine and red leaf lettuces in significant quantities.

Table 5.1 shows that calcium can be found in notable amounts in some fruits, vegetables, nuts, and seeds. Particularly rich sources among these foods include sesame and poppy seeds.

**Table 5.1.** Calcium content of various raw foods

| Food | Calories (kcal) | Calcium (mg) |
|---|---|---|
| **Cabbage family** | | |
| Kale, 3 c (201 g) | 100 | 271 |
| Bok choy, 3 c (210 g) | 27 | 220 |
| Napa cabbage, 3 c (255 g) | 45 | 180 |
| Mustard greens, 3 c (168 g) | 44 | 173 |
| Collard greens, 3 c (108 g) | 32 | 157 |
| Broccoli, florets and stalks, 3 c (273 g) | 93 | 128 |
| Watercress, 3 c (102 g) | 11 | 122 |
| Arugula, 3 c (60 g) | 15 | 96 |
| Cauliflower, chopped, 3 c (321 g) | 80 | 71 |
| **Sunflower family** | | |
| Dandelion greens, 4 c (220 g) | 99 | 411 |
| Romaine lettuce, 1 head (626 g) | 106 | 207 |
| Red leaf lettuce, 1 head (309 g) | 49 | 102 |
| Escarole, 3 c (150 g) | 26 | 78 |
| Romaine lettuce, 4 c (188 g) | 32 | 62 |
| Red leaf lettuce, 4 c (112 g) | 18 | 37 |
| **Other good raw food sources** | | |
| Sesame seeds, whole unroasted, ¼ c (36 g) | 206 | 351 |
| Poppy seeds, 2 Tbsp (17 g) | 88 | 242 |
| Almonds, ½ c (71.5 g) | 411 | 189 |
| Oranges, Valencia, peeled, 2 (242 g) | 119 | 97 |
| Celery, chopped, 2 c (202 g) | 32 | 81 |
| Figs, dried, 5 (42 g) | 105 | 68 |
| Sesame tahini, 1 Tbsp (15 g) | 89 | 63 |

## Calcium Absorption

There are many factors that play important roles in calcium absorption, including vitamin D and boron status. The scientific literature is replete with fascinating studies done on the many concerns surrounding the adequacy of vitamin D, and boron is a mineral easily found on a whole-foods, plant-based diet. We further address vitamin D on pages 100–101.

## Creating Calcium Balance

There are many factors that can cause calcium to be eliminated from the body, so getting enough calcium is not as easy as simply ingesting a particular amount. The delicate dance between factors that help with calcium absorption and those that cause calcium depletion is known as calcium balance.

One substance that causes calcium to be excreted is excess sodium. There are also substances found in foods that may decrease the body's ability to utilize calcium. These include oxalic acid (oxalate) and phytic acid (phytate). (See page 77).

Oxalate in food binds to calcium in food, as well as to other minerals, such as magnesium, iron, and zinc, making the minerals less available to the body. However, oxalate in one food will not inhibit mineral utilization from another food eaten at the same time, nor will it deplete minerals that are already in the body. Research is mixed on the effect of cooking on oxalate. Cooking can have somewhat of an ameliorating effect on oxalate binding, helping to make the calcium in high-oxalate foods more bioavailable. Boiling has a greater effect on oxalate loss than steaming.

It's preferable not to count on high-oxalate foods, such as those in table 5.2, as a main source of calcium in a raw diet, but rather to focus on foods that are lower in oxalate and high in calcium. This doesn't mean that spinach, beet greens, and other high-oxalate foods are not nutritious. They actually contain many other important nutrients besides calcium, such as beta-carotene and vitamin K. Just be sure to get plenty of the foods in table 5.1 that are lower in oxalates as well.

**Table 5.2.** Selected high-oxalate foods per 3.5 ounces (100 g)

| Source | Calories (kcal) | Amount of oxalic acid (mg) |
| --- | --- | --- |
| Parsley, 1⅔ cups | 36 | 1,700 |
| Chives, 1 cup | 30 | 1,480 |
| Purslane, 2⅓ cups | 16 | 1,310 |
| Amaranth, ½ cup uncooked | 371 | 1,090 |
| Spinach, 3⅓ cups | 23 | 970 |
| Beet greens, 2⅔ cups | 22 | 610 |
| Rhubarb, raw, ⅘ cup | 21 | 275–1,336 |

# Iron

In addition to several other important functions, iron is intrinsically involved in the transport of oxygen from the lungs to the cells via the hemoglobin found in red blood cells. The DRI for iron is 8 milligrams for men and postmenopausal women, and 18 milligrams for women who have not reached menopause. Despite the abundance of iron in many whole plant foods, "Where do you get your iron?" is one of the most frequent questions students ask me.

## Sources of Iron

There are several key factors that can influence how well iron can be utilized by the body. The first and most obvious consideration is the iron content of the food eaten. Table 5.3 gives the iron content of a variety of plant foods that are popular among raw-food enthusiasts.

## Different Forms of Iron

The second consideration is the type of iron present in the food. The two main forms of dietary iron are heme iron and nonheme iron. Of these two, heme iron is the primary form found in animal foods, most notably in red meat. Nonheme iron is the form primarily found in plant foods. In popular nutrition literature, I often see concern about getting enough iron from plant-based diets, because of the perception that we absorb more iron from animal foods than plant foods or that heme iron is thought to be better absorbed than nonheme iron.

The reality is more involved than this perception would imply. Nonheme iron is more selectively absorbed than heme iron, helping the body to maintain proper iron balance. The body absorbs more iron from plant foods when the body needs it, such as when iron stores are low, and absorbs less from plant foods when iron stores are higher. Heme iron tends to be absorbed regardless of an individual's iron status.

The most reliable way to know if iron intake is adequate and being utilized properly is to have iron levels and other relevant tests analyzed by a qualified health care provider. One of the issues a blood test can reveal is anemia, a condition characterized by decreased oxygen delivery to cells, resulting in fatigue and other health concerns. A primary cause of anemia is a lack of iron, better known as iron-deficiency anemia. If iron from plant foods was poorly absorbed, vegetarians would have higher incidences of iron-deficiency anemia than omnivores, but this is not the case. Studies have shown that vegetarians don't have any greater incidence of iron deficiency than omnivores.

**Table 5.3.** Iron content of selected raw foods

| Food | Calories (kcal) | Iron (mg) |
|---|---|---|
| **Cabbage family** | | |
| Kale, 3 c (201 g) | 100 | 3.4 |
| Mustard greens, 3 c (168 g) | 44 | 2.5 |
| Broccoli, florets and stalks, 3 c (273 g) | 93 | 2 |
| Bok choy, 3 c (210 g) | 27 | 1.7 |
| Cauliflower, chopped, 3 c (321 g) | 80 | 1.4 |
| **Sunflower family** | | |
| Dandelion greens, 4 c (220 g) | 99 | 6.8 |
| Romaine lettuce, 1 head (626 g) | 106 | 6.1 |
| Red leaf lettuce, 1 head (309 g) | 49 | 3.7 |
| Sunflower seeds, raw, ½ c (70 g) | 409 | 3.7 |
| Romaine lettuce, 4 c (188 g) | 32 | 1.8 |
| Red leaf lettuce, 4 c (112 g) | 18 | 1.3 |
| Escarole, 3 c (150 g) | 25 | 1.2 |
| **Other good raw food sources** | | |
| Sesame seeds, raw, ¼ c (36 g) | 206 | 5.2 |
| Pumpkin seeds, ¼ c (35 g) | 187 | 5 |
| Spirulina, 2 Tbsp (14 g) | 41 | 4 |
| Hemp seeds, 2 Tbsp (20 g) | 113 | 2.4 |
| Cashews, raw, ¼ c (33 g) | 180 | 2.2 |
| Poppy seeds, 2 Tbsp (17 g) | 88 | 1.6 |
| Almonds, ¼ c (36 g) | 206 | 1.3 |

## Proper Iron Balance

In addition to its role in oxygen delivery to cells, iron is also important for energy production, the function of various enzymes, and in DNA synthesis. Iron also has the ability to accept or donate electrons, which can lead to the production of free radicals, which are molecules with missing electrons that can cause damage to proteins, fats, and DNA. This attribute categorizes iron as a prooxidant, the opposite of an antioxidant. So it's important to get enough iron, but not more than necessary. More is not always better! Maintaining proper balance is key.

People who eat plant-based diets obtain all their iron from plant foods. When all or most of their foods are whole plant foods that are naturally high in antioxidants, this helps to offset the prooxidant potential of iron. Omnivores, who generally eat smaller quantities of whole plant foods, may not get the same level of protection, as they may absorb more iron but fewer antioxidants to inhibit iron's prooxidant potential.

People who have trouble absorbing iron and become deficient should consider a dietary change and/or supplement routine that ensures they can absorb the iron they need. This will usually require the assistance of a qualified health care professional who can utilize their knowledge of lab testing, foods, and supplements to be sure the desired results are obtained without putting the person at risk of increased free radical damage.

**Table 5.4.** The phytate content of various plant foods

| Food (100 g dry weight) | Amount of phytate (mg) |
|---|---|
| Wild rice | 2,200 |
| Brazil nuts | 1,719 |
| Sesame seeds | 1,440 |
| Almonds | 1,138 |
| Walnuts | 982 |
| Adzuki beans | 860 |
| Cashews | 630–1,970 |
| Chickpeas | 560 |
| Avocado | 510 |
| Lentils, unsoaked | 440–500 |
| Coconut meat, dried | 357 |
| Dates | 140 |
| Mango | 140 |
| Strawberry | 130 |
| Carrots, raw | 90 |
| Chinese cabbage | 80 |
| Cucumbers, raw | 50 |
| Cauliflower, raw | 50 |
| Tomato | 40–310 |
| Lettuce, romaine | 40 |
| Kale, raw | 13 |
| Spinach, raw | 10–70 |

*Sources:* Data from Macfarlane et al. (1988); Mate and Radomir. (2002); Reddy and Sathe (2001).

## Iron Absorption

The third consideration is the presence of dietary factors that enhance or inhibit iron absorption. The same inhibitors that block calcium, oxalic acid (oxalate) and phytic acid (phytate), also inhibit iron uptake. Researchers of a study published in the *American Journal of Clinical Nutrition* in 2010 found that phytate can play a role in the inhibition of iron absorption in plant-based diets. Phytate is found in a variety of plant foods, such as legumes, grains, nuts, and seeds, and the researchers noted that it's important to focus on foods that are low in phytate.

Table 5.4 shows that fruits and vegetables tend to have lower phytate content than the same weight of nuts, seeds, legumes, and grains. Iron can still be absorbed from these foods, but preparation methods that employ cooking, soaking, germination, and fermentation will help break down phytate, allowing the iron they contain to be more easily absorbed. Note that some legumes in their raw and sprouted form, such as kidney beans, are not recommended and should not be consumed because of the presence of problematic substances, such as phytohemagglutinin, which can lead to gastrointestinal illness.

Soaking and sprouting activates the enzyme phytase in nuts, seeds, grains, and legumes, which breaks down phytate. Soaking may also decrease phytate through the leaching of phytate into the soak water. Table 5.5 shows the results of a study that compared the difference in the available iron in unsoaked, soaked, and sprouted sorghum grain. Soaking and sprouting certainly appeared to make a significant difference, and other available research mirrors these findings.

**Table 5.5.** Processing and iron availability

| Type of sorghum grain | Iron availability (%) |
| --- | --- |
| Raw unsoaked | 8–13.6 |
| Soaked | 14.6–20.8 |
| Germinated | 16.7–20.6 |

*Source:* Data from Afify et al. (2001).

On the other side of the balance equation, vitamin C helps to make the nonheme iron in plant foods more absorbable by converting it to heme iron. It also helps overcome the effects from decreased absorption of phytate and other inhibitors. Many raw foods are excellent sources of vitamin C (see page 95), and combining them in the same meal with foods high in iron can increase their effectiveness. A great example would be a fruit smoothie that includes oranges, strawberries, and iron-rich greens. The greens themselves are also high in vitamin C. It's interesting to note that cooking can break down both phytates and vitamin C. Looking at how cooking high-phytate foods affects iron absorption, it appears that the loss of vitamin C from cooking is at least partially compensated for by the breakdown of phytates.

If phytate and other inhibitors actually had a considerable effect on iron absorption, we'd probably see a much greater prevalence of iron-deficiency anemia within the plant-based community. The fact is, iron-deficiency anemia is not prevalent; nevertheless, the issue shouldn't be ignored, particularly if someone is experiencing low iron status. The preferred approach is to find a diet that works best for a particular individual, given their current circumstances and what's sustainable for them over the long term. Focusing on fruits and meaningful quantities of vegetables is an excellent general strategy for most people.

**Table 5.6.** Magnesium content of various plant foods

| Source | Calories (kcal) | Magnesium (mg) |
|---|---|---|
| Leafy greens | | |
| Romaine lettuce, 1 head (626 g) | 106 | 82.4 |
| Dandelion greens, 4 c (220 g) | 99 | 79.2 |
| Kale, 3 c (201 g) | 100 | 68.3 |
| Bok choy, 3 c (210 g) | 27 | 39.9 |
| Romaine lettuce, 4 c (188 g) | 32 | 26.3 |
| Fruits | | |
| Bananas, 1 medium (118 g) | 105 | 31.9 |
| Oranges, Valencia, peeled, 2 (242 g) | 119 | 24.2 |
| Strawberries, 1 c (166 g) | 53 | 21.6 |
| Mango, 1 whole (207 g) | 135 | 18.6 |
| Other popular raw foods | | |
| Pumpkin seeds, ¼ c (35 g) | 187 | 184.6 |
| Sesame seeds, whole unroasted, ¼ c (36 g) | 206 | 126.4 |
| Sunflower seeds, raw, ¼ c (35 g) | 205 | 113.8 |
| Almonds, ¼ c (36 g) | 206 | 95.8 |
| Cashews, raw, ¼ c (33 g) | 180 | 94.9 |
| Quinoa, uncooked, ¼ c (42.5 g) | 157 | 83.7 |
| Lentils, uncooked, ¼ c (48 g) | 170 | 58.6 |
| Avocado, 1 medium (201 g) | 322 | 58.3 |

## Magnesium

Magnesium plays important roles in the formation of bones and teeth, the activation of over 300 enzymes (including those involved in the production of energy), calcium metabolism, and DNA synthesis. Magnesium is the central atom in the chlorophyll molecule, making leafy green vegetables rich sources of magnesium.

Additional raw plant sources of magnesium include other vegetables, green sprouts, some fruits, and various nuts and seeds. The RDA for magnesium from food sources is 310 to 320 milligrams per day for women and 400 to 420 milligrams per day for men.

Pumpkin seeds are an especially rich source of magnesium, and bok choy is one of the richest sources among the leafy greens. Comparatively, fruit has less magnesium per calorie than other foods listed in table 5.6. However, fruit can be a reliable source of magnesium for followers of a high-sweet fruit raw diet, depending on the type of fruit eaten and the quantity.

---

## Chlorophyll as a Health Food

Chlorophyll is touted as having numerous health benefits—as an antioxidant, blood builder, and a good source of magnesium. These claims may have some credibility, considering that the central atom of the chlorophyll molecule is magnesium, and the chlorophyll molecule has many structural similarities to the human heme molecule that makes up hemoglobin, which is found in red blood cells.

In order for the blood-building claim to hold up, chlorophyll has to be converted to heme in the body. It must be able to survive the digestive system and be absorbed into the bloodstream. Then it has to travel to an area of the body where it can be converted to heme. Finally, there must be enzymes or conversion factors present that can actually make the necessary changes to the chlorophyll molecule to become heme. A lot of things have to function perfectly!

There may be a stronger case for chlorophyll as a magnesium source. Researchers from Ohio State University, Purdue University, the University of North Carolina, and Brown University found that when chlorophyll was digested, magnesium was liberated from the chlorophyll molecule as chlorophyll was broken down into derivatives called pheophytins. (Pheophytins are similar in structure to chlorophyll but contain a hydrogen atom instead of a magnesium atom at the center of the molecule.) The free magnesium was then available to be absorbed by the body. Looking for the presence of pheophytin in the blood after a chlorophyll-rich meal may indicate whether magnesium has been released.

Thus far, only test-tube studies have been done to determine whether these chlorophyll by-products might be absorbed in the intestine, so little is known at this time. But now that researchers know about pheophytins, these substances could become the focus of future studies on whether or not chlorophyll is an antioxidant or can be converted to heme in the human body.

## Potassium

Potassium is involved in muscle contraction throughout the body, including muscles that allow the heart to beat, move food through the digestive tract, and facilitate movement of the skeleton. It also plays an essential role in acid-alkaline balance, especially in the cells and bloodstream (see page 85). While sodium increases urinary excretion of calcium (see page 81), potassium, on the other hand, has the opposite effect, helping the body retain calcium. The adequate intake of potassium for adults is 4,700 milligrams per day.

### Sources of Potassium

Bananas have a reputation for being a great source of potassium, but many other fruits and vegetables are even more abundant sources of this important mineral. Potassium is very easily obtained from numerous plant foods, as shown in table 5.7.

People often express concern about getting too much potassium on plant-based diets, but at this time, there is no established upper limit for potassium, given that intakes of large amounts have not yet been studied in healthy individuals. The IOM does mention that in the absence of an upper limit, caution should be used when exceeding suggested intakes.

We know many people (ourselves included) who have been basing their diets on fruits and vegetables for many decades, and to our knowledge they're not suffering from potassium overload. Overloads and imbalances of nutrients tend to occur when artificially concentrated sources of nutrients, such as poorly designed or improperly used supplements, are taken. Generally, whole foods, such as fruits and vegetables, tend to have abundant yet properly balanced nutrient profiles.

## Sodium

Sodium is an essential mineral that's used by the body for many important processes, including the preservation of fluid balance. In the late 1980s, the National Research Council suggested an intake of 500 mg of sodium per day for adults. A current upper limit of 2,300 mg is suggested by the

**Table 5.7.** Potassium content of various plant foods

| Food | Calories (kcal) | Potassium (mg) |
|---|---|---|
| Honeydew melon, 1 (1 kg) | 360 | 2,280 |
| Cantaloupe, 1 (552 g) | 188 | 1,474 |
| Kale, 3 c (201 g) | 100 | 898 |
| Dandelion greens, 4 c (220 g) | 99 | 873 |
| Papaya, 1 medium (304 g) | 119 | 781 |
| Dates, medjool, 4 pitted (96 g) | 266 | 668 |
| Pomegranate, 1 (282 g) | 234 | 665 |
| Peaches, 2 medium (300 g) | 117 | 570 |
| Celery, chopped, 2 c (202 g) | 32 | 525 |
| Oranges, Valencia, 2 (242 g) | 119 | 433 |
| Apricots, fresh, 1 c, sliced (165 g) | 72 | 427 |
| Tomatoes, chopped, 1 c (180 g) | 32 | 427 |
| Bananas, 1 (118 g) | 105 | 422 |
| Carrots, grated, 1 c (110 g) | 45 | 352 |
| Mango, 1 (207 g) | 135 | 323 |
| Figs, 5 dried (42 g) | 105 | 286 |
| Strawberries, 1 c (166 g) | 53 | 254 |
| Blackberries, 1 c (144 g) | 62 | 233 |

US Department of Health and Human Services (HHS), the IOM, Harvard Health Publications, and the National Academy of Sciences, to name a few. However, in 2010, the upper limit of 2,300 milligrams was reduced to 1,500 milligrams for a significant portion of the US population, including individuals with high blood pressure. The current DRIs for sodium are 1,500 mg for adults up to and including 50 years, 1,300 mg for adults 51 to 70 years, and 1,200 mg over 70 years of age.

The upper limit of 2,300 milligrams for the remaining portion of the US population was established because consumption of sodium in excess of this value is associated with calcium loss in the urine. The scientific community recognizes that the kidneys require the use of calcium to excrete excess sodium. The Centers for Disease Control reported that the average intake of sodium in the United States from 2005 to 2006 was 3,436 milligrams per day, which is largely due to the consumption of processed foods.

Nutrient analyses of different types of raw food diets show a sodium content ranging from 300 to 500 milligrams, providing someone is eating whole, raw plant foods with no added salt or salt products. In analyzing the lab work of many of our raw vegan patients who fit this dietary profile, we have observed this level of sodium to be adequate for many, but not all. We encourage people to be mindful of their sodium intake. Whole food sources of sodium include celery, Swiss chard, and bok choy, all of which can easily provide a notable amount, as indicated in table 5.8. Note that sodium content can add up quickly if salt is used. Even including ¼ teaspoon of salt or salty condiments can add 392 to 590 milligrams of sodium to the diet. It's always best to check the label of any processed product to find the sodium content, if you consume any of these foods. Some natural salt products contain other minerals in addition to sodium, and sodium content among these products can vary. I don't necessarily suggest the consumption of salt products or salty condiments, but I've provided a few in table 5.8 for comparison.

**Table 5.8.** Sodium content of various plant foods

| Food | Calories (kcal) | Sodium (mg) |
| --- | --- | --- |
| Tamari, 1 tsp (6 g) | 3.6 | 335 |
| Nama shoyu, 1 tsp (5 g) | 3.3 | 240 |
| Swiss chard, 3 c (108 g) | 20.5 | 230 |
| Miso, 1 tsp (5.73 g) | 11.4 | 214 |
| Celery, chopped, 2 c (202 g) | 32 | 162 |
| Bok choy, 3 c (210 g) | 27 | 137 |
| Kale, 3 c (201 g) | 100 | 86 |
| Carrots, grated, 1 c (110 g) | 45 | 76 |
| Romaine lettuce, 1 head (626 g) | 106 | 47 |
| Kelp powder, 2 Tbsp (10 g) | 4 | 23 |

## Selenium

Selenium is known for its important and essential role in thyroid function. It also plays a role in the conversion of certain free radicals to water, which in the process restores antioxidant capacity to a molecule produced by our body known glutathione. I've heard people say that selenium itself is an antioxidant, but more specifically, it's needed to help the antioxidant glutathione do its job properly.

The RDA for selenium is 55 micrograms for adults, with an upper limit of 400 micrograms per day. The selenium content of foods varies greatly with the amount of selenium in the soil where the food is grown. One of the richest food sources of selenium is Brazil nuts, provided that they've been grown in selenium-rich soil. According to the USDA nutrient database, one 4.75-gram Brazil nut contains 90.6 micrograms of selenium, which is approximately

165 percent of the RDA for selenium. I typically have a few Brazil nuts per week (but I refrain from eating them by the handful). Vegetables, fruits, sea vegetables, spirulina, and chlorella are not significant sources of selenium. Table 5.9 shows that other nuts and seeds are not significant sources of selenium unless eaten in larger quantities than most raw-food enthusiasts consume. I'm not suggesting that someone eat these foods in such large amounts, as I realize their fat content is high. I include these examples for comparison to show how rich Brazil nuts are as a selenium source versus other nuts and seeds. As with other important nutrients, appropriate lab work analyzed by a properly qualified clinician can determine your selenium status.

**Table 5.9.** Selenium content of various plant foods

| Food | Calories (kcal) | Selenium (mcg) |
|---|---|---|
| Brazil nuts, raw, 4 (19 g) | 124 | 362 |
| Brazil nut, raw, 1 (4.75 g) | 31 | 90.6 |
| Sunflower seeds, raw, ¼ c (35 g) | 205 | 18.6 |
| Amaranth, uncooked, ½ c (96 g) | 358 | 18 |
| Cashews, raw, ½ c (65 g) | 359 | 13 |
| Sesame seeds, raw, ¼ c (36 g) | 206 | 2.1 |

**Table 5.10.** Zinc content of various plant foods

| Food | Calories (kcal) | Zinc (mg) |
|---|---|---|
| Sesame seeds, raw, ¼ c (36 g) | 206 | 2.8 |
| Pumpkin seeds, ¼ c (32 g) | 180 | 2.5 |
| Wild rice, ¼ c (40 g) | 286 | 2.4 |
| Lentils, uncooked, ¼ c (48 g) | 170 | 2.3 |
| Pine nuts, ¼ c (34 g) | 227 | 2.2 |
| Cashews, raw, ¼ c (33 g) | 180 | 1.9 |
| Sunflower seeds, raw, ¼ c (35 g) | 205 | 1.8 |
| Romaine lettuce, 1 head (626 g) | 106 | 1.4 |
| Poppy seeds, 2 Tbsp (18 g) | 92 | 1.4 |
| Almonds, ¼ c (36 g) | 206 | 1.1 |

## Zinc

Zinc is essential for the activity of numerous enzymes in the human body. In addition, zinc plays important roles in cell division, DNA formation, and immune system function. Zinc also is involved in the ability to taste. Good plant sources of zinc include pumpkin seeds, sesame seeds, wild rice, almonds, sunflower seeds, pine nuts, and poppy seeds. The RDAs of zinc for adult women and men are 8 milligrams and 11 milligrams, respectively.

The zinc content of plant-based diets can be lower than omnivorous diets, so knowing rich plant sources of zinc is important for anyone eating a plant-based diet. Soaking and sprouting nuts, seeds, grains, and legumes increases the bioavailability of zinc and other minerals, since these processes break down the phytate found in many foods rich in zinc.

## Copper
Copper is an essential mineral that's involved in many processes in the human body, including the formation of red blood cells, absorption of iron, free radical protection, strengthening of connective tissue, and energy production. The DRI for copper is currently 900 micrograms for both women and men. The raw and plant-based menu plans shown in chapter 10 contain amounts of copper that exceed the DRI, but are not greater than the upper limit of 10,000 micrograms.

## Manganese
Manganese is an essential mineral that's involved in wound healing; bone and cartilage development; antioxidant function; metabolism of carbohydrates, protein, and cholesterol; and other processes. The DRI for manganese is currently 1.8 milligrams for women and 2.3 milligrams for men. The raw and plant-based menu plans shown in chapter 10 contain manganese amounts in excess of the DRI, but not more than the upper limit of 11 milligrams.

## Raw Diets and pH Balance
Minerals play an important role in balancing acid and alkaline substances in the body. Acid and alkaline levels are measured by their pH, a scale that ranges from 0 to 14, with 0 being the most acid and 14 being the most alkaline (basic). A pH of 7.0 is neutral; substances with a pH below 7.0 are acid, while those with a pH above 7.0 are alkaline.

The pH of human blood is slightly alkaline. It ranges from 7.35 to 7.45, with an average of 7.4. This delicate pH range is very tightly regulated.

**Figure 5.1.** The pH of human blood ranges from 7.35 to 7.45

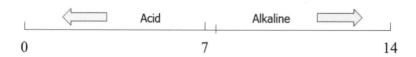

0                              7                              14

The pH on the inside of individual cells in the body averages about 7.0 and is regulated just as tightly as blood pH. This small but important difference in pH between the blood and cells is critical for the exchange of nutrients, waste products, oxygen, and carbon dioxide. Without this regulation of pH, rates of chemical reactions would be altered, enzymes would lose function, proteins would break down, and life itself would not be sustainable.

Because pH balance is so critical to survival, the body has numerous buffering mechanisms to maintain this balance, including the rate of respiration, what's excreted in the urine, and other important mechanisms. A study of 22,034 adult men and women published in the *British Journal of Nutrition* found that diets with higher fruit and vegetable intakes and lower meat intakes were associated with more alkaline urine than diets with lower fruit and vegetable intakes and higher meat consumption. In addition, researchers believe calcium from the skeleton has a role in maintaining acid-alkaline balance.

Scientists at the Research Institute of Child Nutrition in Germany measured the acid-alkaline excretion associated with certain types of foods. Foods associated with net acid excretion in urine have been referred to as acid forming, while foods associated with net alkaline excretion have been referred to as alkaline forming. All foods are some combination of minerals and a variety of other nutrients, and these researchers found that foods rich in calcium, potassium, and magnesium are associated with net alkaline excretion, while foods rich in phosphorus, sulfur, and chloride are associated with net acid excretion. Most fruits are rich in potassium. Leafy greens, among other plant foods, are a rich source of magnesium and often calcium. As stated earlier in this chapter, magnesium is the central atom in the chlorophyll molecule, and green plants, especially leafy greens, are rich in chlorophyll. To summarize, in general, fruits and vegetables are alkaline forming, while most other foods tend to be acid forming to varying degrees. This is particularly true of high-protein animal products, as they contain higher levels of the sulfur-containing amino acids cysteine and methionine than comparable amounts of plant protein.

A number of studies have proposed that increased consumption of fruits and vegetables can have a positive effect on bone health. A 2008 British study published in the *Journal of Nutrition* found that adult men and women consuming a diet high in potassium and other alkaline minerals, such as those found in fruits and vegetables, for one month was associated with greater bone preservation when compared to people who consumed fewer foods containing these minerals. Other research, including the DASH (Dietary Approaches to Stopping Hypertension) studies, as well as in the results of the Framingham

Osteoporosis Study, showed that diets rich in magnesium and potassium from fruits and vegetables were positively associated with greater bone density over four years. Consuming foods rich in these alkaline minerals may decrease the need for the use of calcium from the bones to neutralize excess acid generated by dietary or metabolic factors. Additional research suggests that other nutrients found in fruits and vegetables, such as vitamins K and C and beta-carotene, may play supportive roles in maintaining bone health.

In addition, if people are replacing acid-forming foods in their diet with alkaline-forming fruits and vegetables, there is less acid generated by the diet and simultaneously a higher intake of alkaline-forming minerals. This is positive for both mineral and pH balance.

## CHAPTER 6

# Vitamins

⎯⎯⎯⎯⎯ ∞∞∞ ⎯⎯⎯⎯⎯

A VITAMIN IS A NUTRIENT THAT IS ESSENTIAL for the proper functioning of an organism, including growth, metabolism, and maintenance of health. Vitamins don't provide calories, but are important for numerous functions, including the conversion of carbohydrate, protein, and fat into energy.

There are two main classifications of vitamins: water-soluble and fat-soluble. The classifications are defined by how the vitamins are best absorbed, whether or not the body can store them, where they are used, and what potential the vitamins have for toxicity if consumed in excess.

## Water-Soluble Vitamins

Water-soluble vitamins are found primarily in watery portions of the body, such as the bloodstream, and are best absorbed in the presence of water. They include vitamin C and the B-complex vitamins. Water-soluble vitamins are generally not stored by the body, so it's important to get the necessary amount of these vitamins every day. A notable exception is vitamin $B_{12}$, a water-soluble B vitamin that can be stored in the liver. When excess amounts of water-soluble vitamins are consumed, the body simply excretes what's not needed, so there's little risk of getting a toxic dose.

### Vitamin $B_{12}$ (Cobalamin)

Vitamin $B_{12}$ has many important functions in the body. It's involved with the synthesis of DNA, functioning of the nervous system, helping to keep homocysteine levels appropriately low in the bloodstream, the formation of red blood cells, and in energy production. Vitamin $B_{12}$ is created by certain species of bacteria. It can be made by bacteria in the large intestine, but unfortunately $B_{12}$ is absorbed in the last part of small intestine (the distal ileum) prior to reaching the large intestine. $B_{12}$ is also the one vitamin that can be difficult, if not impossible, to obtain on a raw vegan diet, so we give it particular attention here.

There are many signs and symptoms of vitamin $B_{12}$ deficiency, but I suggest supplementing this vitally important nutrient in adequate amounts on a regular basis before symptoms of deficiency are noticeable. At that point, irreversible conditions may already have developed. Vitamin $B_{12}$ insufficiency and deficiency may occur in vegans or raw foodists who don't supplement or consume $B_{12}$-fortified foods, given that plant foods are not a reliable source.

It's important to note that vitamin $B_{12}$ deficiency is not unique to people who consume a plant-based diet. Researchers in the Framingham Offspring Study found that 39 percent of the almost 3,000 people studied could be classified as insufficient or deficient in $B_{12}$. These people were not vegans or even raw-food vegans—they were omnivores. This study provides evidence that an omnivorous diet does not guarantee good $B_{12}$ status.

Spirulina, sea vegetables, and fermented foods were once thought to be reliable sources of vitamin $B_{12}$, but they were since found to contain $B_{12}$ analogs, molecules that can bind to $B_{12}$ receptors in the body but don't have the same effect on the body as human bioactive $B_{12}$. Research published in the *American Journal of Clinical Nutrition, Annals of Nutrition and Metabolism, International Journal for Vitamin and Nutrition Research*, and *Experimental Biology and Medicine* indicates that these foods are now seen as unreliable sources of $B_{12}$.

There are two forms of vitamin $B_{12}$ that are active in the human body: methylcobalamin and adenosylcobalamin. Sixty to 80 percent of the cobalamin in the blood is in the form of methylcobalamin, while up to 20 percent is adenosylcobalamin. Supplemental forms of vitamin $B_{12}$ that I have seen include methylcobalamin, hydroxocobalamin, cyanocobalamin, and cobalamin. Since it's one of the primary bioactive forms of $B_{12}$, methylcobalamin is absorbed and used as is by the body. Hydroxocobalamin, cyanocobalamin, and cobalamin can be absorbed and converted by the body into the forms necessary for metabolic function. I personally use methylcobalamin supplements and have experienced good results with this form of $B_{12}$.

The Dietary Reference Intake (DRI) for vitamin $B_{12}$ is currently 2.4 micrograms for both women and men. The DRI for adult pregnancy is 2.6 micrograms. Typical amounts in $B_{12}$ supplements tend to range from 500 to 1,000 micrograms and sometimes less in multivitamins. Why so much in these supplements? Some people may have trouble absorbing vitamin $B_{12}$ for various reasons, and the hope is that the person will absorb some percentage of what they ingest and the net effect will be adequate $B_{12}$ absorption. Fortunately, since vitamin $B_{12}$ is a water-soluble vitamin, the potential for toxicity is thought to be low. Whatever amount the body doesn't use can be stored in the liver or various other tissues in small amounts or simply excreted.

Supplements provide adequate levels for the majority of people, but I'm in favor of $B_{12}$ testing to know for sure if someone is getting enough from supplements—whether they eat a plant-based diet or not. $B_{12}$ injections are another option, especially for people who may have trouble absorbing oral doses. There are several lab tests that we use in our practice to measure $B_{12}$ status, including serum $B_{12}$, serum and urinary methylmalonic acid

(MMA), serum homocysteine, hemoglobin, hematocrit, red blood cell count, and mean corpuscular volume (MCV). Each one of these tests tells part of the picture, and educated clinicians can utilize one or a number of them to determine $B_{12}$ status. Check with an appropriately qualified health care provider to get reliable information on $B_{12}$, $B_{12}$ testing options, and supplementation recommendations.

### Vitamin $B_1$ (Thiamin, Thiamine)

Thiamin plays a very important role in the conversion of carbohydrates to energy, an example of why B vitamins have been referred to as the "energy Bs."

Thiamin can be found in a number of raw plant foods, with nuts and seeds being some of the richest sources, along with fruits and vegetables, especially leafy greens. Grains, including millet, and pseudograins, such as quinoa and amaranth, are good sources of thiamin. Many raw-food enthusiasts soak and sprout quinoa before eating, while some who eat cooked foods will cook grains and pseudograins before eating them. We've observed that thiamin status can be significant in raw-food enthusiasts who consume large amounts of produce. In other words, it all adds up!

The DRIs for thiamin are 1.1 milligrams for women and 1.2 milligrams for men. The DRI for adult pregnancy is 1.4 milligrams.

**Table 6.1.** Selected plant sources of thiamin

| Source | Calories (kcal) | Thiamin (mg) |
|---|---|---|
| Sunflower seeds, raw, ½ c (70 g) | 409 | 1.04 |
| Dandelion greens, 4 c (220 g) | 99 | 0.42 |
| Pine nuts, ¼ c (33.8 g) | 227 | 0.42 |
| Millet, uncooked, ½ c dry (100 g) | 378 | 0.42 |
| Romaine lettuce, 1 head (626 g) | 106 | 0.42 |
| Brown rice, medium-grain, ½ c dry (95 g) | 356 | 0.32 |
| Quinoa, raw, ½ c dry (85 g) | 313 | 0.31 |
| Sesame seeds, unroasted, ¼ c (36 g) | 206 | 0.28 |
| Cashews, raw, ½ c (65 g) | 359 | 0.27 |
| Kale, 3 c (201 g) | 100 | 0.22 |

### Vitamin $B_2$ (Riboflavin)

Like thiamin, riboflavin plays an important role in producing energy from carbohydrates and fat. Riboflavin is also involved in the metabolism and activation of other nutrients, such as vitamin $B_6$, vitamin A, and folate. It indirectly helps keep cells from being damaged by free radicals, because of its role in regenerating the antioxidant glutathione.

The DRIs for riboflavin are 1.1 milligrams for women and 1.3 milligrams for men. The DRI for adult pregnancy is 1.4 milligrams. Excess consumption of riboflavin, especially from some supplements, may result in bright yellow urine. Riboflavin has many of the same food sources as thiamin.

**Table 6.2.** Selected plant sources of riboflavin

| Source | Calories (kcal) | Riboflavin (mg) |
|---|---|---|
| Almonds, ½ c (71.5 g) | 411 | 0.73 |
| Romaine lettuce, 1 head (626 g) | 106 | 0.39 |
| Buckwheat, uncooked, ½ c dry (85 g) | 292 | 0.36 |
| Millet, uncooked, ½ c dry (100 g) | 378 | 0.29 |
| Quinoa, uncooked, ½ c (85 g) | 313 | 0.27 |
| Avocado, 1 med. (201 g) | 322 | 0.26 |
| Sunflower seeds, raw, ½ c (70 g) | 409 | 0.25 |
| Kale, 3 c (201 g) | 100 | 0.22 |
| Wild rice, ½ c dry (80 g) | 286 | 0.21 |
| Amaranth, ½ c dry (96 g) | 358 | 0.19 |

## Vitamin B₃ (Niacin)

Niacin is involved in energy production and is important for both the synthesis and breakdown of fat. It plays an essential role in the manufacture of cholesterol and cholesterol-based hormones, including estrogen, progesterone, testosterone, and cortisol. Niacin helps with the formation of 7-dehydrocholesterol, which is important for vitamin D production in the skin. Table 6.3 shows selected plant sources of niacin, including legumes, grains, and pseudograins. Some raw-food enthusiasts soak and sprout buckwheat and lentils before eating them, while some who eat cooked foods will cook grains, legumes, and pseudograins (such as brown rice, lentils, and quinoa) before eating them. The DRIs for niacin are 14 milligrams for women and 16 milligrams for men. The DRI for adult pregnancy is 18 milligrams.

## Vitamin B₅ (Pantothenic acid)

Pantothenic acid is another B vitamin that plays a critical role in energy production, specifically the processing of carbohydrates, protein, and fat for energy. It's also a component of coenzyme A (CoA), which is important for many cellular functions such as the manufacture of red blood cells. The DRI for pantothenic acid is 5 milligrams for both women and men. The DRI for adult pregnancy is 6 milligrams.

**Table 6.3.** Selected plant sources of niacin

| Source | Calories (kcal) | Niacin (mg) |
|---|---|---|
| Buckwheat, ½ c dry (85 g) | 292 | 5.97 |
| Sunflower seeds, raw, ½ c (70 g) | 409 | 5.83 |
| Wild rice, ½ c dry (80 g) | 286 | 5.39 |
| Brown rice, medium-grain, ½ c dry (95 g) | 356 | 4.23 |
| Avocado, 1 medium (201 g) | 322 | 3.49 |
| Lentils, sprouted, 2 c (235 g) | 249 | 2.65* |
| Lentils, ½ c dry* (96 g) | 339 | 2.50 |
| Almonds, ½ c (71.5 g) | 411 | 2.42 |
| Kale, 3 c (201 g) | 100 | 2.01 |
| Romaine lettuce, 1 head (626 g) | 106 | 1.84 |
| Sesame seeds, raw, ¼ c (36 g) | 206 | 1.63 |

* One-half cup of dry lentils becomes 2 cups sprouted lentils after soaking for eight hours and sprouting for about two days. In lentils, the niacin content increases with soaking and sprouting, but the calorie content decreases, which is likely due to the calories being used to fuel the growth of the sprout.

**Table 6.4.** Selected plant sources of pantothenic acid

| Source | Calories (kcal) | Pantothenic acid (mg) |
|---|---|---|
| Avocado, 1 medium (201 g) | 322 | 2.79 |
| Cauliflower, 3 c (321 g) | 80 | 2.09 |
| Broccoli, florets and stalks, 3 c (273 g) | 93 | 1.51 |
| Amaranth, ½ c dry (96 g) | 358 | 1.41 |
| Lentils, sprouted, 2 c (235 g) | 249 | 1.36 |
| Buckwheat, ½ c dry (85 g) | 292 | 1.05 |
| Wild rice, ½ c dry (80 g) | 286 | 0.86 |
| Romaine lettuce, 1 head (626 g) | 106 | 0.84 |
| Cashews, raw, ½ c (65 g) | 359 | 0.56 |
| Bananas, 1 medium (118 g) | 105 | 0.39 |

## Vitamin $B_6$ (Pyridoxine)

Pyridoxine plays a very important role in the formation of proteins used in the body for structural and functional purposes and is essential for the synthesis of serotonin and dopamine (brain neurochemicals), histamine (important in immune system responses), heme (a major component of red blood cells), and taurine (a nonessential amino acid). When glycogen, the form of glucose stored in the liver and muscles, is broken down to make energy, pyridoxine plays a very important role in this conversion.

The DRI for pyridoxine is 1.3 milligrams for both women and men up to and including age 50. The DRIs for women and men age 51 and over are 1.5 milligrams and 1.7 milligrams, respectively. The DRI for adult pregnancy is 1.9 milligrams.

**Table 6.5.** Selected plant sources of pyridoxine

| Source | Calories (kcal) | Pyridoxine (mg) |
|---|---|---|
| Cauliflower, 3 c (321 g) | 80 | 0.71 |
| Amaranth, ½ c (96 g) | 358 | 0.57 |
| Dandelion greens, 4 c (220 g) | 99 | 0.55 |
| Kale, 3 c (201 g) | 100 | 0.54 |
| Avocado, 1 medium (201 g) | 322 | 0.52 |
| Broccoli, florets and stalks, 3 c (273 g) | 93 | 0.46 |
| Lentils, sprouted raw, 2 c (235 g) | 249 | 0.45 |
| Romaine lettuce, 1 head (626 g) | 106 | 0.44 |
| Bananas, 1 medium (118 g) | 105 | 0.43 |
| Red bell pepper, chopped, 1 c (149 g) | 46 | 0.43 |
| Bok choy, 3 c (210 g) | 27 | 0.41 |

### Vitamin B₇ (Biotin, also known as vitamin H)

Biotin is involved in the production of energy from carbohydrates and some proteins and in the synthesis of fatty acids. When more calories are consumed than the body needs, excess carbohydrates can be stored as glycogen in the liver and muscles or can be transformed into body fat. Biotin is involved in both of these processes when it helps with the liberation of glucose from glycogen and plays a role in the formation of fatty acids. Biotin is also important for the breakdown of the amino acids leucine, isoleucine, threonine, and methionine when they are needed to generate energy.

The DRI for biotin is 30 micrograms for both women and men. The DRI for adult pregnancy is 30 micrograms.

### Vitamin B₉ (Folate or folic acid)

The word folate is derived from the Latin word for foliage, which makes sense given that some strong sources of folate are leafy greens. Folate is the form of this vitamin found in whole foods, while folic acid is the form found in supplements and fortified foods. Along with vitamin B$_{12}$, folate is critical for cell division and DNA replication and decreases blood levels of homocysteine, a substance associated with inflammation. Folate is susceptible to damage from heat, so in general, raw foods tend to be higher in folate content than their cooked counterparts.

The DRI for folate is 400 micrograms for both women and men. The DRI for adult pregnancy is 600 micrograms.

**Table 6.6.** Selected plant sources of biotin

| Source | Calories (kcal) | Biotin (mcg) |
|---|---|---|
| Almonds, ½ c (71.5 g) | 411 | 45.8 |
| Peanuts, raw, ⅓ c (48.7 g) | 276 | 35 |
| Romaine lettuce, 1 head (626 g) | 106 | 11.2 |
| Avocado, 1 medium (201 g) | 322 | 7.2 |
| Cauliflower, 3 c (321 g) | 80 | 4.8 |
| Sesame seeds, unroasted, ¼ c (36 g) | 206 | 4 |
| Raspberries, 1 c (123 g) | 64 | 2.3 |
| Romaine lettuce, 4 c (188 g) | 32 | 3.6 |
| Bananas, 1 medium (118 g) | 105 | 3.1 |
| Kale, 3 c (201 g) | 100 | 1.01 |

**Table 6.7.** Selected plant sources of folate

| Source | Calories (kcal) | Folate (mcg) |
|---|---|---|
| Romaine lettuce, 1 head (626 g) | 106 | 800.3 |
| Spinach, 1 bunch (340 g) | 78 | 659.6 |
| Romaine lettuce, 4 c (188 g) | 32 | 255.7 |
| Cauliflower, 3 c (321 g) | 80 | 183 |
| Collard greens, 3 c (108 g) | 32 | 179.3 |
| Broccoli, florets and stalks, 3 c (273 g) | 93 | 166.3 |
| Avocado, 1 medium (201 g) | 322 | 162.8 |
| Quinoa, ½ c dry (85 g) | 313 | 156.4 |
| Bok choy, 3 c (210 g) | 27 | 138.6 |
| Papaya, 1 medium (304 g) | 119 | 115.5 |
| Oranges, Valencia, 2 peeled (242 g) | 119 | 94.4 |
| Dandelion greens, 4 c (220 g) | 99 | 59.4 |
| Kale, 3 c (201 g) | 100 | 58.3 |

## Choline

Choline is generally recognized as a member of the B-vitamin family and is manufactured by the body from the amino acids methionine and serine. It's used to make acetylcholine, a neurotransmitter responsible for a variety of functions in the brain and elsewhere in the body. Choline can be recycled in the nervous system, and apparently this recycling mechanism is the richest source of choline used in the creation of acetylcholine. Choline is also involved in memory and is used to make phosphatidylcholine and sphingomyelin, important parts of cell membranes.

The DRIs for choline are 425 milligrams for women and 550 milligrams for men. The DRI for adult pregnancy is 450 milligrams. Although choline can be manufactured from certain amino acids, it's considered to be an essential nutrient that needs to be acquired through diet or supplements.

**Table 6.8.** Selected plant sources of choline

| Source | Calories (kcal) | Choline (mg) |
|---|---|---|
| Cauliflower, 3 c (321 g) | 80 | 145.1 |
| Mung beans, ½ c dry (104 g) | 359 | 101.3 |
| Lentils, ½ c dry (96 g) | 339 | 92.5 |
| Amaranth, ½ c dry (96 g) | 358 | 67.4 |
| Spinach, 1 bunch (340 g) | 78 | 61.2 |
| Quinoa, ½ c dry (85 g) | 313 | 59.7 |
| Broccoli, florets and stalks, 3 c (273 g) | 93 | 49.4 |
| Soy lecithin, 1 Tbsp (14 g) | 103 | 47.3 |
| Almonds, ½ c (71.5 g) | 411 | 37.3 |
| Avocado, 1 medium (201 g) | 322 | 28.5 |
| Collard greens, 3 c (108 g) | 32 | 25.1 |

On several occasions, I've heard raw-food educators say that cauliflower looks like the human brain, so it must be a good brain food. I always found this to be funny. However, looking at these numbers, I now wonder if cauliflower just might be a brain food after all.

## Vitamin C

Vitamin C has numerous functions in the body, one of the most important being its antioxidant activity. It also helps in the formation of collagen, found in bone, skin, gums, and the lining of blood vessels. In the skin, for example, collagen helps maintain strength and elasticity. When collagen is damaged, wrinkles may result. Vitamin C acts not only to help collagen form properly in the first place, but also helps keep free radicals from causing damage to collagen after its formation.

Vitamin C is extremely easy to find on a raw food diet. The DRIs for vitamin C are 75 milligrams for women and 90 milligrams for men. The DRI for pregnant adult women is 85 milligrams. Note that the DRIs for vitamin C are the minimum intakes needed to avoid scurvy, a vitamin C deficiency. The optimal amounts of vitamin C are likely higher. Fortunately, the amount of fruits and vegetables consumed by many raw-food enthusiasts provide amounts of vitamin C well above the DRI.

**Table 6.9.** Selected plant sources of vitamin C

| Source | Calories (kcal) | Vitamin C (mg) |
|---|---|---|
| Camu camu, pulp, 100 g* | Not reported | 864–3,000 |
| Acerola cherry, fresh, 1 c (98 g) | 31.36 | 1,644 |
| Kale, 3 c (201 g) | 100 | 241.2 |
| Red bell pepper, chopped, 1 c (149 g) | 46 | 190.3 |
| Romaine lettuce, 1 head (626 g) | 106 | 141.2 |
| Oranges, Valencia, 2 (242 g) | 119 | 117.4 |
| Strawberries, 1 c (166 g) | 53 | 97.6 |
| Spinach, 1 bunch (340 g) | 78 | 95.5 |
| Dandelion greens, 4 c (220 g) | 99 | 77 |

* *Sources:* Data from Justi et al. (2000); Nascimento et al. (2013).

Leafy greens and many types of fruit are the richest sources of vitamin C. Camu camu (*Myrciaria dubia*) is a fruit native to the Amazon rainforest in Brazil that has become a popular so-called superfood, based on its significant vitamin C content. Since vitamin C is a water-soluble vitamin, it can be lost in cooking water when foods are processed or heated. However, studies done at the State University of Campinas and the State University of Maring, both in Brazil, found that even after processing, camu camu retains a notable amount of vitamin C, an amount greater than that in many fruits and vegetables.

Raw-food enthusiasts who consume a large percentage of their calories from fruits and vegetables already consume an amount of vitamin C well in excess of the daily value. The consumption of alleged superfoods high in vitamin C is entirely optional and likely not additionally helpful on diets that already provide significant amounts.

## Fat-Soluble Vitamins

Fat-soluble vitamins are found in fatty areas of the body and cell membranes. They include vitamin A and other carotenoids, vitamin D, vitamin E, and vitamin K. Unlike most water-soluble vitamins, fat-soluble vitamins can be stored by the body. When they're consumed in excess amounts, the body may experience toxic effects, depending on the vitamin. A good example of this is vitamin A toxicity from excess vitamin A intake, which may lead to birth defects and other serious conditions.

There's a built-in regulation mechanism in plant foods that helps one avoid excess vitamin A intake. A good example of this regulator is the carotenoid beta-carotene. Beta-carotene is a precursor to vitamin A and will only form vitamin A when the body needs it. It's found in plant foods, while vitamin A is found in animal foods. Even though the body can store beta-carotene in large amounts, beta-carotene appears on the Food and Drug Administration's "Generally Recognized as Safe" list, since one study found that even 180 milligrams of beta-carotene ingested daily produced no serious side effects (other than giving the skin a yellow or orange cast). My personal diet averages about 54 milligrams (54,000 micrograms) per day, which is what naturally occurs in the fruits and vegetables I consume.

### Vitamin A (Retinol)

Vitamin A is essential for proper cell growth and reproduction and is probably best known for its importance in maintaining vision. It also plays an important role in immune system function and skin health.

Vitamin A is found exclusively in animal foods. Vegans do not obtain vitamin A directly from plant foods, but instead consume compounds known as carotenoids, some of which can be converted to a form of vitamin A known as retinol. These carotenoids are found abundantly in specific fruits and vegetables. They have yellow, orange, and red coloring and are well known for their antioxidant activity. The carotenoids that can be converted to vitamin A (called pro-vitamin A carotenoids) are beta-carotene, alpha-carotene, gamma-carotene, and beta-cryptoxanthin.

Since the body converts only a portion of pro-vitamin A carotenoids into the retinol form of vitamin A, a system to measure conversion, known as retinol activity equivalent (RAE), is used to measure how much vitamin A can be converted from carotenoids in a food or supplement, if needed. The resulting vitamin A is expressed in micrograms of RAE. Table 6.10 compares the proportions of the various pro-vitamin A carotenoids found in foods that can be converted to retinol.

**Table 6.10.** The conversion rate of pro-vitamin A carotenoids to RAE

| Nutrient | Proportion converted to RAE |
|---|---|
| Beta-carotene, dissolved in oil | ½ |
| Beta-carotene, common dietary | 1/12 |
| Alpha-carotene, common dietary | 1/24 |
| Gamma-carotene, common dietary | 1/24 |
| Beta-cryptoxanthin, common dietary | 1/24 |

*Source:* Data from Hendler and Rorvik (2008).

Of the carotenoids, beta-carotene has the greatest vitamin A activity. The body converts beta-carotene into retinal (a precursor to retinol) by splitting the beta-carotene molecule in half. Retinal is then converted into retinol. Carotenoids that aren't converted to retinol can be stored in fat cells throughout the body.

People who consume large amounts of fruits and vegetables high in carotenoids may develop an orange color to their skin, which may be indicative of carotenoids being stored in fat cells in the skin. Vitamin A itself is stored in the liver, and when the liver reaches its capacity, toxicity, or hypervitaminosis A, occurs. However, neither beta-carotene nor any of the other carotenoids lead to toxicity, so this orange coloring is only cosmetic and doesn't indicate liver problems or other issues as has been rumored. A study reported in the 1990s identified health challenges in male Finnish smokers associated with the consumption of synthetic beta-carotene derived from supplements. However, a study published in the *American Journal of Clinical Nutrition* reported that none of those issues have been identified with consumption of the beta-carotene naturally occurring in fruits and vegetables.

Given that carotenoids are fat-soluble, it's generally understood that they're best absorbed in the presence of fat. Therefore, the consumption of nuts, seeds, or avocado with vegetables, in the form of a nut-based dressing, for example, may allow for greater absorption of carotenoids.

The DRIs for vitamin A (as retinol and RAE) are 700 micrograms for adult women and 900 micrograms for adult men. The DRI for vitamin A in pregnancy is 770 micrograms. The tolerable upper intake levels for vitamin A in women, men, and pregnant women is 3,000 micrograms.

More about Carotenoids

Carotenoids that aren't converted to vitamin A also have significant nutritional functions. Lutein and zeaxanthin are yellow carotenoids that function synergistically and play an important role in vision. They function as antioxidants and may keep the macula, a disk-shaped structure in the back of the eyeball, from being damaged by UVB spectrum rays of the sun. Researchers are in the process of determining the role of lutein and zeaxanthin in macular health and if they potentially have a role in protection from macular degeneration.

**Table 6.11.** Selected plant sources of beta-carotene and their RAE

| Source | Calories (kcal) | Beta-carotene (mcg) | RAE |
|---|---|---|---|
| Romaine lettuce, 1 head (626 g) | 106 | 30,752 | 2,563 |
| Kale, 3 c (201 g) | 100 | 18,544 | 1,545 |
| Dandelion greens, 4 c (220 g) | 99 | 12,879 | 1,118 |
| Cantaloupe, 1 (552 g) | 188 | 11,150 | 933 |
| Yam, 1 (130 g) | 112 | 11,062 | 922 |
| Carrots, grated, 1 c (110 g) | 45 | 9,114 | 919 |
| Romaine lettuce, 4 c (188 g) | 32 | 9,825 | 819 |
| Butternut squash, cubed, 1 c (140 g) | 63 | 5,916 | 744 |
| Green leaf lettuce, 4 c (144 g) | 22 | 6,398 | 533 |
| Bok choy, 3 c (210 g) | 27 | 5,630 | 469 |
| Red leaf lettuce, 4 c (112 g) | 18 | 5,034 | 420 |
| Collard greens, 3 c (108 g) | 32 | 4,149 | 360 |
| Red bell pepper, chopped, 1 c (149 g) | 46 | 2,420 | 233 |
| Papaya, 1 medium (304 g) | 119 | 839 | 166 |
| Apricots, fresh, sliced, 1 c (165 g) | 72 | 1,805 | 159 |
| Mango, 1 (207 g) | 135 | 921 | 80 |
| Tomatoes, chopped, 1 c (180 g) | 32 | 808 | 75 |

Lycopene is a red carotenoid with antioxidant activity that's found in a small number of foods, including red tomatoes and tomato products. There is currently no established daily value for lycopene, but a group of researchers at the University of Toronto suggests an intake of 35 milligrams per day.

The amount of lycopene present in tomatoes can vary significantly depending on the color and cultivated variety. Given that lycopene is a red pigment, generally the more red pigment contained in the tomato, the greater the lycopene content. A study done at Heinrich Heine University Düsseldorf in Germany reported that the reddest strains of tomatoes tested had 50 milligrams of lycopene per kilogram, while yellow tomatoes had 5 milligrams of lycopene per kilogram.

**Table 6.12.** Selected plant sources of lutein and zeaxanthin

| Source | Calories (kcal) | Lutein and zeaxan-thin (mcg) |
|---|---|---|
| Kale, 3 c (201 g) | 100 | 79,496 |
| Dandelion greens, 4 c (220 g) | 99 | 29,942 |
| Romaine lettuce, 1 head (626 g) | 106 | 13,605 |
| Collard greens, 3 c (108 g) | 32 | 9,647 |
| Romaine lettuce, 4 c (188 g) | 32 | 4,347 |
| Summer squash, chopped, 2 c (226 g) | 36 | 4,802 |
| Broccoli, florets and stalks, 3 c (273 g) | 93 | 3,704 |
| Green leaf lettuce, 4 c (144 g) | 22 | 2,491 |
| Red leaf lettuce, 4 c (112 g) | 18 | 1,931 |
| Carrots, grated, 1 c (110 g) | 45 | 282 |
| Papaya, 1 medium (304 g) | 119 | 228 |

As a carotenoid, lycopene is fat-soluble and is best absorbed when the form of a food is highest in fat and lowest in water. When a food is dried, it becomes more concentrated, and its nutrients become more concentrated as well. Similarly, when water is removed from a tomato, the lycopene content becomes more concentrated. Sun-dried tomatoes have a particularly high lycopene content, as shown in table 6.13.

**Table 6.13.** Selected plant sources of lycopene

| Food | Lycopene content (mg/100 g) |
|---|---|
| Sun-dried red tomatoes | 45.9 |
| Tomato paste | 28.8 |
| Tomato sauce | 13.9 |
| Tomato ketchup | 12.1 |
| Tomato juice | 9.7 |
| Guava | 5.2 |
| Watermelon | 4.5 |
| Tomatoes, raw red | 2.6 |
| Papaya | 1.8 |
| Pink grapefruit | 1.4 |

It's often thought that lycopene can be better absorbed from cooked tomatoes than raw tomatoes. A review of the scientific literature published in the journal *Cancer Epidemiology, Biomarkers and Prevention* surveyed 23 lycopene studies and found that the absorption of lycopene had more to do with the concentration of lycopene relative to water and concentration of fat relative to water than with any other aspect of cooking. As lycopene concentration and fat concentration rose, absorption of lycopene increased. These two factors can also be achieved with dehydration. We have yet to know whether more lycopene is absorbed from dehydrated raw foods than water-rich raw foods, since no studies have been done at this time. I also look forward to a study that compares the absorption of lycopene from raw dehydrated foods versus cooked foods. In the meantime, when I make a dressing that includes tomatoes and or sun-dried tomatoes, I add some avocado and or chia seeds, which may help with lycopene absorption.

**Vitamin D**
Vitamin D plays a very important role in bone health and the maintenance of blood calcium levels. Recently, it's been studied for its role in the possible prevention of various health challenges, including autoimmune diseases, certain types of cancer, and infectious diseases.

Vitamin D has been called the sunshine vitamin because when sunlight hits the skin, it interacts with 7-dehydrocholesterol to produce cholecalciferol (vitamin $D_3$). Cholecalciferol is then transformed by the liver into 25-hydroxycholecalciferol, also known as 25-hydroxyvitamin $D_3$. Then 25-hydroxycholecalciferol travels to the kidneys, where it's transformed to 1,25-dihydroxycholecalciferol, or 1,25-dihydroxyvitamin $D_3$, which is considered to be the activated or hormonal form of vitamin D. Vitamin D is a fat-soluble vitamin, but sun exposure has not been found to produce vitamin D toxicity.

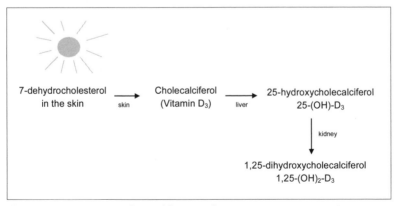

**Figure 6.1.** Vitamin D is obtained from supplements or sun exposure

How much vitamin D can the skin make? This is dependent upon a number of factors, including the amount of cloud cover, pollution, sunscreen usage, latitude, season, skin tone, length of exposure, areas of body exposed, time of day, and age. Overhead sun in the spring, summer, and fall seasons is optimal, with summer being the best time of year for vitamin D production. It's true that sunscreen can inhibit the production of vitamin D, but many researchers encourage people to use sunscreen or curtail their exposure to the sun because of skin cancer concerns. SPF 8 sunscreen can block up to 95 percent of the production of vitamin D in the skin.

People living at 35 degrees north latitude (southern California and North Carolina) or below were found to produce vitamin D in their skin year-round, while people living north of 35 degrees did not produce vitamin D in the winter. People living in Canada, the northern United States, northern Europe, southern South America, southern Australia, and New Zealand may not make enough vitamin D for their needs during the winter months. Apparently, the sun's rays in these areas are more oblique and not as powerful in the winter months. This is also true in the early morning and late afternoon in the spring, summer, and fall. For the same amount of exposure, people with fair skin tend to produce more vitamin D than people who have darker skin, since darker skin contains more melanin, which blocks the ability of ultraviolet rays to enter the skin. Given all the factors that can affect the ability of the skin to make vitamin D from the sun, it can be challenging to determine how much sun exposure is appropriate without going overboard. I have found the sun exposure charts in the book *The Vitamin D Solution* (Plume, 2010) written by Michael Holick, PhD, MD, to be very helpful in determining how much sun exposure is appropriate for any skin type.

The RDA for vitamin D is measured in international units; for adults the RDA is 600 IU and for adults over 70 years old, it's 800 IU. Some clinicians and researchers don't agree with these recommendations, given the widespread incidence of vitamin D insufficiency and deficiency in Western society, and would like to see the recommendations increased.

Supplemental forms of vitamin D are vitamin $D_3$ and vitamin $D_2$. Vitamin $D_2$ is sourced from vegetarian ingredients. The best way to know if your vitamin D supplement is working or if you are experiencing a vitamin D insufficiency or deficiency is to get a vitamin D test. Supplementation options should be considered with the help of an experienced and qualified health care practitioner.

## Vitamin E

As an antioxidant and fat-soluble nutrient, vitamin E plays a very important role in protecting cell membranes from free radicals, specifically the polyunsaturated fats that comprise cell membranes. It's also been studied for possible benefits for heart health, since it's been found to decrease the oxidation of LDL cholesterol, which may help prevent the formation of arterial plaque.

Vitamin E is a family of compounds consisting of two classes; tocopherols and tocotrienols. Each class has four individual vitamin E compounds known as vitamers. Of these vitamers, alpha-tocopherol has the greatest vitamin E activity, followed by beta-, gamma-, and delta-tocopherol. Alpha-tocopherol has been considered the vitamin E standard against which all the other vitamers are measured, but in recent years compelling research has been done at Rutgers University on the activity of gamma- and delta-tocopherols.

Given that vitamin E is fat-soluble, it's plentiful in fatty plant foods. Vitamin E has been found to have less potential for toxicity than vitamin A; however, there have been some reported adverse events from consumption of large doses of vitamin E supplements. The DRI for vitamin E is 15 milligrams for women, men, and pregnancy.

There's generally less vitamin E in animal foods than plant foods. (In table 6.14, beef is listed for comparison purposes.) In comparing red leaf lettuce to beef, for example, one serving of each contains 0.46 milligrams of vitamin E. However, the beef has almost six times more calories. This means that per calorie, red leaf lettuce has nearly six times more vitamin E than beef!

**Table 6.14.** Selected plant sources of vitamin E

| Source | Calories (kcal) | Vitamin E (mg) |
|---|---|---|
| Sunflower seeds, raw, ½ c (70 g) | 409 | 23.3 |
| Almonds, ½ c (71.5 g) | 411 | 18.8 |
| Dandelion greens, 4 c (220 g) | 99 | 7.6 |
| Avocado, 1 medium (201 g) | 322 | 4.2 |
| Collard greens, 3 c (108 g) | 32 | 2.4 |
| Red bell pepper, chopped, 1 c (149 g) | 46 | 2.4 |
| Quinoa, ½ c dry (85 g) | 313 | 2.1 |
| Broccoli, florets and stalks, 3 c (273 g) | 93 | 2.1 |
| Amaranth, ½ c dry (96 g) | 358 | 1.2 |
| Tomatoes, chopped, 1 c (180 g) | 32 | 1 |
| Romaine lettuce, 1 head (626 g) | 106 | 0.8 |
| Red leaf lettuce, 1 head (309 g) | 49 | 0.5 |
| Beef, 80% lean, 4 oz (113 g) | 288 | 0.5 |

## Vitamin K

Vitamin K has two natural forms: vitamin $K_1$ and vitamin $K_2$. Vitamin $K_1$, also known as phylloquinone, plays an important role in blood clotting and bone health. Good sources of vitamin $K_1$ include leafy green vegetables. Vitamin $K_2$, also known as menaquinone, has been studied for its function in bone health.

Vitamin $K_2$ has several forms; the two for which I've seen the most research are menaquinone-4 and menaquinone-7. There have been some concerns about getting enough vitamin $K_2$, specifically menaquinone-4, on a plant-based diet. Researchers at Tohoku University and Kobe Pharmaceutical University in Japan noted that the conversion of vitamin $K_1$ to vitamin $K_2$ (specifically menaquinone-4) has been demonstrated in mice and rats, but the potential for this conversion has yet to be fully understood in humans. In addition, a University of Maastricht study noted that $K_1$ can be converted by bacteria in the GI tract of humans into menaquinone-7. Vitamin $K_2$ appears to be absorbed in the last part of the small intestine and the large intestine, but specifics on the absorption of vitamin $K_2$ are still under investigation.

The DRIs for vitamin K are 90 micrograms for women and 120 micrograms for men. The DRI for pregnancy is 90 micrograms.

**Table 6.15.** Selected plant sources of vitamin $K_1$

| Source | Calories (kcal) | Vitamin K1 (mcg) |
|---|---|---|
| Dandelion greens, 4 c (220 g) | 99 | 1,712 |
| Kale, 3 c (201 g) | 100 | 1,642 |
| Spinach, 1 bunch (340 g) | 78 | 1,642 |
| Romaine lettuce, 1 head (626 g) | 106 | 603 |
| Collard greens, 3 c (108 g) | 32 | 552 |
| Broccoli, florets and stalks, 3 c (273 g) | 93 | 268 |
| Watercress, 3 c (102 g) | 11 | 255 |
| Romaine lettuce, 4 c (188 g) | 32 | 193 |
| Bok choy, 3 c (210 g) | 27 | 96 |

# CHAPTER 7
# Water and Hydration

——— ∽∽∽ ———

A N IMPORTANT AND OFTEN-OVERLOOKED health consideration is
hydration. Water is involved in many essential body processes and
makes up a significant percentage of body weight. How much water should
be consumed and in what form?

The Institute of Medicine has set adequate intakes (AIs) for water consumption based on median intakes by healthy individuals who are adequate-
ly hydrated, shown in table 7.1. These AIs are for people living in temperate
climates, and they don't take into account exercise, perspiration, sodium
intake, humidity, and several other factors, all of which may alter the amount
of water needed for adequate hydration. Nevertheless, the AIs do give us
something to go on. Maybe of most importance, the recommendations take
into account not only what we consume from drinking water and other bever-
ages directly, but also (and I want to stress) from food.

**Table 7.1.** The daily water AIs for adults 19 years and older

|  | Milliliters/liters | Ounces | Quarts |
|---|---|---|---|
| Men | 3,700/3.7 | 125 | approximately 4 |
| Women | 2,700/2.7 | 91 | approximately 3 |

The amount of water that can be found in foods varies greatly depending on the food and how it's prepared. Fresh fruits and vegetables can have
a high water content, whereas nuts, seeds, and dehydrated or dried foods,
such as dried fruits, may be less water-rich. If a food is steamed or boiled,
that process may increase its water content; think of uncooked oatmeal or
brown rice versus cooked. If a food has been baked, roasted, or broiled, it
may have lost water content.

To compare the water content found in a variety of raw menus, refer to
the menus listed in chapter 10. The high-sweet fruit menu consisting of 2,000
calories (kcal) on page 131 contains 4,181 milliliters of water (over 1 gallon)
and exceeds the AIs for both women and men. Unless someone lives in a hot
and dry climate, is physically active outdoors, perspires a lot, or consumes
a significant amount of salt, it's likely that they would be well hydrated from
the foods in this menu.

A similar menu on page 133 with just over 3,000 calories contains 4,943 milliliters of water, which is nearly 5 liters (just over 5 quarts). Many people who choose to consume a high-sweet fruit raw diet are also very physically active and need more calories. When fruits and vegetables are chosen, those extra calories also come with plenty of extra water, replacing what was lost with activity.

Another approach to raw food involves eating much smaller amounts of sweet fruit. The low-sweet fruit menu on page 135 contains only 1,773 milliliters of water, which is much less water than that found in the previous menu plans. Calorie-wise, this menu is most similar to the 2,051-calorie high-sweet fruit menu, which contains 4,181 milliliters of water. Why such a big difference in water content between these two raw menus? First of all, fruit generally tends to be very water rich unless it's dried or very concentrated (as with dates). Secondly, nuts and seeds are much less water rich than fruits, and the high amount of nuts and seeds in this menu would change the proportions of water content. If nuts and seeds are soaked, their water content will increase. The water content of this menu was measured using unsoaked nuts and seeds. With a low-sweet fruit menu, a substantial amount of additional water will likely need to be included.

Many raw-food enthusiasts eat a diet in between a high-sweet fruit or low-sweet fruit diet, and an intermediate raw diet is given on page 138. Not surprisingly, the water content is somewhere between the two previous approaches and exceeds the daily AI for water in women. In addition, some raw-food enthusiasts, including Dr. Rick and me, occasionally add some cooked foods to their diet, and on page 141 there's a menu plan that includes 80 percent raw foods and 20 percent cooked foods. This 80-percent raw menu actually provides more water (2,532 milliliters) than the 100-percent raw low-sweet fruit menu (1,773 milliliters) for a similar number of calories (about 2,000). Even with some cooked food, a predominately raw menu such as this one can provide a large amount of the daily AI for water. The amount of water in these sample menus may vary significantly depending on the foods eaten. The more nuts, seeds, oils, and dehydrated foods in a diet, the less water there will be. Fresh fruits and vegetables and their juices contribute far more water to the diet than most cooked and processed foods. Soaked nuts and seeds obviously contain more water than their unsoaked counterparts, but are still much lower in water than fresh fruits and vegetables.

**Table 7.2.** Selected plant foods and their water content

| Food | Water content (ml) |
|---|---|
| **Fruits** | |
| Apple, medium (182 g) | 156 |
| Avocado, medium (201 g) | 147 |
| Banana, medium (118 g) | 88 |
| Blueberries, 1 c (148 g) | 125 |
| Dates, medjool, pitted, 2 (48 g) | 10 |
| Lemon, medium (84 g) | 75 |
| Mango, medium (207 g) | 169 |
| Orange, Valencia, medium (121 g) | 104 |
| Papaya, medium (304 g) | 270 |
| **Vegetables** | |
| Broccoli, chopped, 2 c (162 g) | 145 |
| Carrot, medium (119 g) | 106 |
| Cucumbers, sliced, 1 c (104 g) | 99 |
| Dandelion greens, 2 c (82 g) | 70 |
| Kale, raw, chopped, 3 c (201 g) | 170 |
| Romaine lettuce, shredded, 7 c (329 g) | 311 |
| Tomatoes, chopped, 1 c (180 g) | 170 |
| Yam, raw, medium (343 g) | 265 |
| Zucchini, chopped, 2 c (218 g) | 206 |
| **Nuts and seeds** | |
| Almonds, raw, ½ c (72 g) | 3.4 |
| Brazil nuts, raw, 3 (14 g) | 0.5 |
| Cashews, raw, ½ c (65 g) | 3.4 |
| Chia seeds, 2 tsp (8.5 g) | 0.4 |
| Coconut oil, unrefined, 1 Tbsp (14 g) | 0 |
| Macadamia nuts, raw, ½ c (67 g) | 0.9 |
| Olive oil, extra virgin, 1 Tbsp (13.5 g) | 0 |
| Pumpkin seeds, raw, ½ c (69 g) | 4.8 |
| Sesame seeds, raw, ½ c (72 g) | 3.4 |
| Sunflower seeds, raw, ½ c (70 g) | 3.3 |

*Source:* Data from Food Processor Nutrition and Fitness Software, ESHA Research, Inc.

In comparison with the predominantly or all-raw menus analyzed previously, let's take a look at a couple of menus based on cooked vegan foods. A day's meals might consist of cooked oatmeal with an apple for breakfast, vegetable soup with a hummus and pita sandwich for lunch, black beans and brown rice with steamed kale and a large (6-cup) salad for dinner, and some figs and raw almonds for a snack. The water content of this menu might come in at 1,700 to 1,800 milliliters, which is much lower than that of the mostly or all-raw food plans, with the exception of the low-sweet fruit menu.

A vegan cooked menu with a higher proportion of raw food might omit the soup and sandwich and include a large raw salad, cooked beans and grains, and a lot of steamed veggies. A typical menu like this might contain 3,000 to 3,500 milliliters of water, approximately double the previous one. Not only do both raw and steamed veggies contain quite a bit of water, but grains will also absorb more water when cooked. One-half cup of uncooked medium-grain brown rice increases in water content from 12 milliliters to 196 milliliters when cooked in one and a half cups of water.

The bread in the pita sandwich mentioned previously contains very little water. Table 7.3 demonstrates how much less water is in various breads, even whole-grain bread, when compared to whole grains cooked in water.

**Table 7.3.** Water content of various breads and brown rice (for comparison)

| Food | Water content (ml) |
|---|---|
| Bread, whole wheat pita, 1 (64 g) | 20 |
| Bread, multigrain, 1 slice (26 g) | 9.6 |
| Bread, white, 1 slice (25 g) | 9.1 |
| Brown rice, medium grain, dry, ½ c (95 g) | 12 |
| Brown rice, medium grain, boiled, 1¾ c (269 g) | 196 |

Finally, the standard Western menu on page 144 contains the least amount of water on any menu plan we have described: 1,329 milliliters. When I compare the DRIs for water (2,700 milliliters for women and 3,700 milliliters for men), I can understand the reason experts suggest that people drink quite a bit of water per day. This menu contains very few vegetables and no fruit, and many of the foods on this plan are quite calorie dense. There's a lesser volume of food in this menu plan in comparison to the other plans, but this smaller amount of food provides almost 2,200 calories. The other menu plans contain a greater volume of food that is lower in calories and higher in water content. Focusing the diet on whole plant foods, with plenty of fruits and vegetables, can help people get the right amount of water and calories (in addition to so much else), while helping them feel full and satisfied.

## CHAPTER 8

# The Effect of Heat on Nutrients and Enzymes

DOES HEAT AFFECT THE NUTRIENT CONTENT OF FOODS? The answer is definitely yes, but it depends on the type of nutrient, cooking temperature, length of cooking time, and to an extent, surface area and volume. Not all nutrients are affected equally by heat.

## Minerals

Research has indicated that individual minerals are not affected by cooking, given that the actual structure of the mineral is not changed by heat. However, the organic matter surrounding the mineral can be affected; therefore, heat can indirectly affect mineral content. This can happen when liquid containing some of the minerals that have leached out of food is drained after cooking. Researchers at the University of Kyoto in Japan found in their study that the content of sodium, potassium, calcium, phosphorus, magnesium, iron, zinc, manganese, and copper in cooked vegetables was on average 60 to 70 percent that of raw vegetables. The greatest mineral loss occurred when foods were boiled in water and then drained. Frying (although not an optimal cooking method for many reasons) resulted in less mineral loss than boiling, while stewing retained the greatest mineral content, as the cooking liquid containing minerals from food was consumed as part of the stew.

Contrary to belief within the raw-food community, cooking may actually help improve the absorption of certain minerals in certain foods. Two examples of substances well known to decrease the absorption of minerals, such as calcium, iron, and zinc, are phytic acid (phytate) and oxalic acid (oxalate). Oxalic acid and phytic acid bind to these minerals, making them unavailable to the body. Numerous studies show that both of these substances are broken down with all types of cooking and steaming, making calcium, iron, and zinc more usable. At the same time, there are other nutrients, such as certain vitamins, that are lost with cooking, so raw plant foods that are low in oxalic acid and phytic acid, such as kale and lettuce, will contain more nutrients than their cooked counterparts.

## Vitamins

Vitamins can be negatively affected not only by heat but also by varying degrees of heat, depending on the type of vitamin and the heating method.

Because water tends to heat up more quickly than fat, water-soluble vitamins tend to be more susceptible to damage from cooking than fat-soluble vitamins. Steaming appears to result in the least amount of vitamin loss, followed by boiling and frying. With steaming, the temperature of the steam rising off the boiling water is 212 degrees F (100 degrees C) and the food is not submerged or directly in contact with the water. With boiling, food is submerged and in direct contact with the water. With frying, food is in direct contact with or submerged in the frying medium, which is usually some type of oil or fat that is generally hotter than boiling water.

A study done by researchers at the University of Parma in Italy examined the effects of steaming, boiling, and frying on vitamin C levels in broccoli florets. Steaming for five minutes resulted in the loss of 32 percent of vitamin C, while 48 percent was lost with boiling, and 87 percent was lost during frying. Researchers at Poznan University in Poland found that steaming broccoli did not change vitamin C levels, while a group of researchers whose study was published in the *Journal of Food Science* found that vitamin C losses when broccoli was steamed or boiled were 22 percent and 34 percent, respectively, for identical cooking times. Given this, there appears to be less vitamin C loss with steaming than with boiling and more vitamin C loss with higher-temperature cooking methods.

Like vitamin C, folate is a water-soluble vitamin and is therefore more susceptible to loss with cooking than fat-soluble vitamins. A study published in the *British Journal of Nutrition* found that more folate is lost with boiling than steaming of broccoli florets. The researchers found that boiling resulted in the following approximate losses:

- 48 percent of folate in 5 minutes
- 56 percent of folate in 10 minutes
- 65 percent of folate in 15 minutes

They also found that steaming broccoli florets for 5 to 15 minutes resulted in no significant decrease in folate and observed a similar trend in spinach leaves. Boiling spinach resulted in the following approximate losses:

- 51 percent of folate in 5 minutes
- 58 percent of folate in 10 minutes
- 68 percent of folate in 15 minutes

Another study, from Royal Veterinary and Agricultural University in Denmark, found that boiling broccoli florets for five minutes resulted in the loss of 45 to 64 percent of folate and vitamin $B_6$, while steaming them for five minutes resulted in the loss of zero to 17 percent of folate and vitamin $B_6$.

Additional research confirms that steaming causes the least amount of vitamin loss compared to other cooking methods. Several researchers agree that vitamins C and $B_1$ and folate are among the nutrients most sensitive to heat, while some B vitamins, such as niacin, biotin, and pantothenic acid, are thought to be more stable when subjected to heat.

Information on vitamin E is varied. Many studies say that very little to no vitamin E is lost with any type of water-based cooking method, which is not surprising given that vitamin E is a fat-soluble vitamin. One study done in Geissen, Germany, compared boiling, stewing, and steaming of broccoli. Cooking the broccoli did not result in a loss of vitamin E, but may have actually made vitamin E more bioavailable. More specifically, no loss of vitamin E was found as the result of the following:

- boiling broccoli florets for 16 minutes
- stewing broccoli florets for 8 minutes
- steaming broccoli florets for 10 minutes

## Raw versus Cooked Vegetables

A 2004 study published in *Cancer Epidemiology, Biomarkers & Prevention* noted that an increase in the consumption of both raw or cooked vegetables was related to a lower incidence of colorectal, esophageal, gastric, lung, oral, and pharyngeal cancers. However, these researchers also said that the effect was significantly stronger for raw vegetables than cooked. They proposed that this may be due to the changes in nutrient availability, destruction of enzymes, and alteration of structure and digestibility of food caused by cooking, but they also said more data is necessary to be conclusive.

Cooking and vitamin loss is not an all-or-nothing situation but more of a continuum, as shown in the previous studies. In addition to nutrient loss, there are other considerations with cooking. In our Science of Raw Food Nutrition classes, we discuss various substances known to have carcinogenic and other negative health effects (acrylamide, advanced glycation end products, nitrosamines, and polycyclic aromatic hydrocarbons, among others) that are formed in particular foods cooked using certain cooking methods. Whether or not these unhealthful substances form or not, and the extent to which they do, depends on a number of factors, including the type of food, cooking temperature, and cooking time. It's good to know that at this point none of these unhealthful substances have been detected when foods are steamed or boiled. Given the lack of problematic substance formation and minimized nutrient loss (as well as maintenance of water content), we see steaming as the most preferred cooking method.

Steaming can be very useful for preparing certain foods that many people find to be difficult to digest raw. A good example is lightly steamed broccoli. Most of the vitamins appear to be retained with steaming, and the broccoli may be easier to digest because the fiber has softened. I believe that all else being equal, the better a food is digested, the more nutrients it will provide. For many people, this increase in digestibility outweighs the relatively minor nutrient loss that occurs with steaming. In addition, it's often easier to consume more steamed vegetables than raw vegetables. If 20 percent of the nutrients in a food are lost through steaming but intake of the food is doubled or tripled, steaming may allow someone to come out way ahead nutritionally.

The bottom line here is that we don't see all cooking as bad. Instead we consider the use of heat on a case-by-case basis. Cooking can certainly have its place when nutritional content, personal preferences, and social factors are taken into account.

## The Effects of Heat on Enzymatic Activity in Food

People are often given bits and pieces of information about enzymes by various raw-food educators and aren't really sure how to put all this disparate information together. This next section provides a solid foundation in traditional enzyme theory and current enzyme research.

### Enzymes Defined

Researchers have learned much about enzymes since they were first identified in the 1800s. Some of this information confirms what those early scientists identified, while some of what has been learned has taken that early knowledge to the next level.

An enzyme is a molecule that catalyzes chemical reactions. An enzyme name generally contains the suffix "ase" in combination with the substance it breaks down, such as the enzyme lactase and the sugar lactose. Enzymes are made of protein, which denatures, or breaks down, at certain temperatures. This is one reason why enzymes are lost with heating. Most enzymes found in food have been shown to break down starting at 104 degrees F (40 degrees C), which is higher than body temperature, although not all enzymes present in a food will be lost the moment this temperature is reached. *The Manual of Clinical Enzyme Measurements* states that the longer a food is heated at temperatures above this threshold, the more enzymes will be lost.

Enzyme inhibitors are found in nuts, seeds (including grains and pseudograins), and legumes. When these foods are soaked in water for several hours, the enzyme inhibitors break down, allowing the enzymes contained in the foods to become activated, often leading to germination (sprouting) and an increase in digestibility.

## Digestive, Metabolic, and Food Enzymes

There are many types of enzymes: those found in foods and plants, as well as enzymes that are part of digestive and metabolic processes in the human body. Digestive enzymes are made in the body and released into the mouth (via saliva), the stomach, and the small intestine (via the pancreas), in response to the consumption of food. The main categories of digestive enzymes made by the body are lipase for fat digestion, amylase for carbohydrate digestion, and protease for protein digestion. Carbohydrate and fat digestion begins in the mouth, as saliva contains salivary amylase and lingual lipase. Protein digestion begins in the stomach with hydrochloric acid, along with pepsin, a protein-digesting enzyme. When food moves from the stomach into the small intestine, the pancreas releases pancreatic lipase, amylase, and proteases. This allows carbohydrate, fat, and protein digestion to continue in the small intestine. The pancreas releases all these enzymes at once, since most foods contain a combination of carbohydrate, fat, and protein. (See table 1.1 on pages 6–7.) The lining of the small intestine also secretes amylase and protease, which further contribute to the digestion of carbohydrate and protein.

Can we run out of digestive enzymes, and if so, are we enzymatically bankrupt for the rest of our lives? The concept of an enzyme "bank account" was proposed by Dr. Edward Howell, who was born in 1898 and graduated from medical school in the early 1900s. More current research makes it clear that the body produces digestive enzymes as needed throughout the life span.

Metabolic enzymes are produced by the body and used to initiate or increase the speed of biochemical reactions within the body. They activate very specific reactions. Plant enzymes are found in plant tissues and have important functions related to the growth and maintenance of life-sustaining processes within plants.

Do the enzymes found in raw plant foods contribute to human digestion? Before answering this question, we must consider the types of enzymes actually found in plants. As mentioned earlier, the human digestive tract secretes carbohydrate-, protein-, and fat-digesting enzymes, known as amylase, protease, and lipase. Plants produce all three categories of these enzymes as well. Plants produce amylases to convert the complex carbohydrate starch into simpler carbohydrates, such as maltose. For example, during the day, a plant makes starch through the process of photosynthesis and then at night, the plant uses amylase to transform the starch into simpler sugars for use in the creation of energy for the plant. Plants also produce proteases, such as the cysteine proteases found in papaya and pineapple. These proteases, known as papain and bromelain, have been shown to digest proteins in the human digestive tract. Lipases are also produced in plants, especially in seeds, where they are used to create energy from fats necessary for the growth of the plant during and after the seed germination process.

To summarize, it is clear that plant enzymes perform essential metabolic activities within plants, and many of these enzymes are involved in carbohydrate, protein, and fat transformation. The degree to which these plant enzymes can contribute to digestion in humans has yet to be fully understood. Any digestive activity of these enzymes would have to take place prior to contact with hydrochloric acid in the stomach, since enzymes are proteins and hydrochloric acid eventually denatures proteins.

## Phytochemical Activation

Certain plant enzymes have been shown to activate particular phytonutrients. A group of researchers at Columbia University found that these enzymes can be denatured by heat, which keeps the phytonutrients from becoming fully active.

One example of a plant enzyme that activates phytonutrients is myrosinase, which is found in raw cruciferous vegetables, such as broccoli, cauliflower, bok choy, collard greens, kale, and other members of the cabbage family. These plants contain beneficial phytonutrients called glucosinolates, which are transformed into other substances by myrosinase. Myrosinase and glucosinolates are embedded in separate cells within plant tissue, so they're only able to interact with each other once plant cells are broken down by some form of cellular disruption, such as chewing, blending, chopping, or juicing. Myrosinase reacts with glucosinolates and the resulting compounds are known as isothiocyanates. Isothiocyanates have antioxidant properties that can help eliminate certain carcinogens through detoxification processes that take place in the liver.

Several studies show that heating cruciferous vegetables reduces the amount of isothiocyanates created, since myrosinase is degraded by the heating process. A study published in *Nutrition and Cancer* showed that steaming broccoli for fifteen minutes inactivated myrosinase to some degree, but not completely. The same study showed the formation of isothiocyanates in the participants who ate the steamed broccoli was one-third the amount of isothiocyanates formed in those who ate the raw broccoli. Because the glucosinolate content of the broccoli was maintained during the steaming process, the logical conclusion was that the lower isothiocyanate levels that resulted after eating steamed broccoli were due to the degradation of myrosinase.

This does not mean that steaming is all bad. The researchers explain that not everyone finds it easy to chew and digest raw broccoli, and since the glucosinolate content was not significantly affected, steaming would be the best choice of cooking method. This same group of researchers found in an earlier study that glucosinolates were significantly reduced when watercress was boiled for three minutes, and myrosinase was also completely inactivated. They also mentioned that microwaving broccoli at full power for eight minutes resulted in considerable loss of sulforaphane, a type of glucosinolate. Given the amount of research currently available, steaming results in the smallest loss of glucosinolates and myrosinase in comparison to other cooking methods.

Alliinase is an enzyme found in garlic that converts another substance in garlic, alliin, into allicin. Allicin is a sulfur-containing compound studied for possible antioxidant and antibacterial properties, among others. Alliin doesn't appear to have the same activity as allicin, so the transformation by alliinase is essential in order for these healthful properties to be realized.

As with myrosinase, alliinase is activated with the disruption of the garlic plant cells, such as when they're crushed or cut. A 2001 study published in the *Journal of Nutrition* showed that microwaving garlic for 60 seconds completely inactivated alliinase activity and boiling garlic at 212 degrees F (100 degrees C) for 20 minutes suppressed antibacterial abilities. This same study showed that subjects exposed to a carcinogen (cancer-causing substance) had a 64 percent reduction in carcinogenic activity after eating raw garlic. After they ate garlic that had been microwaved for 60 seconds or heated in an oven for 45 minutes, protection from this carcinogen was reduced.

Allicin itself is generally thought not to be affected by heat, so chopping garlic and letting it sit for ten minutes on a cutting board allows the alliin and alliinase to interact and form allicin. Even if the chopped or crushed garlic is heated after that, the allicin will remain. If the garlic is heated prior to chopping, the enzyme alliinase will be deactivated and will not be able to convert alliin into allicin.

## In Summary

Not all nutrients are equally affected by heat. Minerals, while not individually affected by heat, can be lost in discarded cooking water. Water-soluble vitamins are generally more readily broken down with certain cooking methods than fat-soluble vitamins, and steaming generally results in loss of fewer water-soluble vitamins than other cooking methods.

Enzymes are proteins and are therefore susceptible to damage by heat. Plant enzymes, such as alliinase and myrosinase, are important for the activation of phytonutrients in garlic and cruciferous vegetables, respectively. The human body creates the digestive enzymes amylase, protease, and lipase for the digestion of carbohydrate, protein, and fat. The degree to which plant amylases, proteases, and lipases can contribute to human digestion has yet to be fully understood.

## CHAPTER 9

# Understanding Calorie Density and Macronutrient Percentages

THE AMOUNT OF ENERGY OBTAINED FROM FOOD is measured in calories. The concept of calorie density compares the relative impact of various foods on calorie consumption by noting the number of calories in similar quantities of foods. The calorie density of a food is the number of calories per measurement of weight, such as calories per gram or calories per pound. The greatest determinants of calorie density are the water, fat, and fiber content of a food. Of these components, water is by far the greatest determinant of calorie density. All else being equal, the more water a food contains, the lower the calorie density of that food. For example, water-rich grapes have fewer calories per pound than raisins. Raisins, with less water than grapes, are more concentrated in calories for the same weight, so are more calorie dense.

The higher the fat content of a food, the higher the calorie density. This is because fat contains over twice as many calories per gram as carbohydrate and protein.

Carbohydrate = 4 calories/gram

Protein = 4 calories/gram

Fat = 9 calories/gram

As a result, high-fat foods will be more calorie dense than their low-fat counterparts.

The higher the fiber content of a food, the lower the calorie density. Fiber, like water, takes up space and contributes to the weight of food but doesn't supply any calories. Because fiber and water add bulk, they dilute calories. Fresh fruits and vegetables are naturally water rich, low in fat, and high in fiber in comparison to concentrated foods that are high in fat and/or contain less water and fiber.

## How to Calculate Macronutrient Percentages

I've seen the percentages of carbohydrate, protein, and fat reported by nutrition professionals and researchers both as a percentage of calories and as a percentage of weight. The reporting of macronutrients in these ways serves different purposes. Looking at them as a percentage of calories is advantageous because it takes into account their calorie content. Components of food that don't make a calorie contribution, including water and fiber, are appropriately not part of the equation. In contrast, food labels report macronutrient content by weight.

Percentage of calories, percentage of weight—does knowing the difference really matter? This difference is often a source of confusion for many people. Knowing how each is calculated can help explain the difference and the significance.

To determine the percentage of calories from carbohydrate, protein, and fat in a food, start by gathering the information on a food label or from an online nutrient analysis website to find the following information about a food or menu plan:

- total weight of the food item in grams
- total calories of the food item (energy and kcal on the USDA Nutrient Database)
- fat content in grams
- protein content in grams
- carbohydrate content in grams

To convert the information in grams to a percentage of calories, refer to the listing on the previous page for the calorie content of the macronutrients. These values may vary depending on the food being analyzed, so using these approximations may not give you exactly the same values that are derived when precise conversion factors are used. However, these average values are very close and for most purposes are close enough.

To get the final result, calculate the following:

- percentage of calories from fat = total fat grams x 9, then divided by the number of total calories and multiplied by 100
- percentage of calories from protein = total protein grams x 4, then divided by the number of total calories and multiplied by 100

The percentage of calories from carbohydrate can be found by subtracting the fat and protein percentages from 100. The percentage of calories from carbohydrate can also be calculated by multiplying total carbohydrate in grams by 4, then dividing by the number of total calories.

Taking avocado as an example, a whole avocado weighs on average 136 grams. It contains 227 calories, has 20.96 grams of fat, 2.67 grams of protein, and 11.75 grams of carbohydrate. (The remaining 100.62 grams consist of water, fiber, and other substances that don't contribute to calories.) Following the bullet points directly above, you'd calculate:

Fat: 20.96 x 9 = 188.64, then divide 188.64 by 227 = 0.83. Multiply 0.83 x 100 = 83%

Protein: 2.67 x 4 = 10.68, then divide 10.68 by 227 = 0.05. Multiply 0.05 x 100 = 5%

Carbohydrate: 100% – 83% – 5% = 12%

The percentage of carbohydrate can also be calculated using this method:

Carbohydrate: 11.75 x 4 = 47.0, then divide 47.0 by 227 = 0.21. Multiply 0.21 x 100 = 21%.

Why the discrepancy in percentages of carbohydrate between the two methods? The complete explanation is technical, multifaceted, and beyond the scope of this book. It's important to note that the 4-4-9 conversion factors for protein, carbohydrate, and fat (often referred to as general Atwater factors) are only averages, and the actual conversion factors (often called specific Atwater factors) can vary by the food being analyzed. For example, specific Atwater factors for carbohydrate in various vegetables can range from 3.7 to 4 calories per gram, in contrast to carbohydrate in raw fruits ranging from 2.5 to 3.6 calories per gram. Specific Atwater factors for protein and fat vary by food as well. Although the more general system isn't perfect, it's easy to use and can give valuable ballpark information on the macronutrient percentages in foods.

To calculate the macronutrient content of an avocado as a percentage of weight, divide the weight of each macronutrient by the total weight of the avocado and multiply each by 100:

Fat: 20.96 divided by 136 = 0.15. Multiply 0.15 x 100 = 15%

Protein: 2.67 divided by 136 = 0.02. Multiply 0.02 x 100 = 2%

Carbohydrate: 11.75 divided by 136 = 0.09. Multiply 0.09 x 100 = 9%

If the nutrients are shown as a percentage of weight, the avocado is shown to be 15 percent fat, 2 percent protein, and 9 percent carbohydrate. This can be misleading, since other components, such as water and fiber, contribute to the weight or volume of a food, but don't make a contribution to calories. When people are considering foods to eat, they are generally interested in how many calories are in the food, not how much it weighs. Looking at the macronutrient content as a percentage of calories gives one a better understanding of the calorie sources within that food and is a better representation of the caloric makeup of that food.

A good example of this would be a combination of oil and water. Oil contains 100 percent of its calories from fat, given that carbohydrate and protein were separated from it during the oil extraction process. If one teaspoon of oil is poured into a glass of water, what percentage of the calories in the oil and water mixture is from fat? Given that water itself does not contain any sources of calories, the mixture contains 100 percent of calories from fat. By weight, the oil may be 5 percent and the water may be 95 percent. Someone who wants to make the water and oil combination appear to be low fat would report that the combination has 5 percent fat, whereas in reality, 100 percent of the calories come from fat. This is how corporations can say that a product is 96 percent fat-free (by weight) when in fact 50 percent of the calories come from fat. As misleading and confusing as it is, this practice is perfectly legal in the United States.

## Applying Calorie Density to Foods and Menus

Researcher and author Barbara Rolls, PhD, championed the concept of calorie density in her book *Volumetrics* (Harper, 2000). She suggested that foods with calorie densities between 272 and 681 calories per pound should make up the majority of a diet if someone is interested in achieving their optimal weight (see table 9.1). This averages out to about 477 calories per pound, so if this is the average calorie density of all the foods eaten in a day, satisfying quantities of those foods should provide the right amount of calories for achieving and maintaining a healthy weight.

**Table 9.1.** The calorie density of various foods and food groups

| Food (average amounts) | Calorie density (calories per pound) |
| --- | --- |
| Raw vegetables | 100 |
| Raw sweet fruits | 200–300 |
| Cooked legumes | 400 |
| Cooked grains | 500 |
| Meat and meat products | 500–2,418 |
| Dairy products | 225–3,275 |
| Avocado | 800 |
| Bread (whole wheat) | 1,135 |
| Sea vegetable, dulse, dry | 1,197 |
| Coconut pulp (mature)* | 1,607 |
| Nuts and seeds | 2,500–2,750 |
| Oil | 4,000 |

* The values for young coconut are not included on this table since reliable, research-based data was not available at the time of publication.

The foods with the lowest calorie density are fresh vegetables and fruits, since these foods contain the most water and are low in fat and high in fiber. If someone were eating only vegetables, they would have to consume 20 pounds of them to obtain 2,000 calories. No matter how excited one gets about eating raw vegetables, the likelihood of consuming all the calories needed exclusively from vegetables is from slim to none!

A real-world example would be the very basic vegetable salad I eat regularly. Ingredients for this salad vary depending on availability. (See page

123.) Without dressing, it weighs almost two pounds. It contains 4 cups of romaine lettuce, 4 cups of chopped dandelion greens or other type of greens, 1 cucumber, 1 large tomato, 1 cup of grated carrot, 1 cup of chopped celery, and ½ cup of chopped fresh basil. This vegetable-only salad (without dressing) is 191 calories. In order to get the 2,000 calories that I need daily from vegetables, I would have to eat over ten of these salads a day! I don't think that would be possible, even given how much I love vegetables.

I'd have to assume that most people would struggle with that many large salads a day, which is why if someone is eating a 100-percent raw vegan diet, they're largely getting their calories from fruit, fat, or both. Fruits are higher in calorie density than vegetables, so meeting one's daily calorie need with fruit is much easier than with vegetables. People who eat a 100-percent high-sweet fruit or low-fat raw diet eat quite a bit of fruit to get enough calories and often emphasize higher-calorie fruits, such as bananas, in their diet.

If someone is eating a 100-percent raw vegan diet without much fruit, the calories will come largely from nuts, seeds, and avocados (which are very calorie dense) or perhaps higher-calorie sprouts, such as lentil or pea sprouts. Sprouted grains and dehydrated sprouted grain crackers can also increase calorie content, but these aren't often used as dietary staples.

Nuts, seeds, and oils are very calorie dense. If people eat a significant amount of them, they may not realize how many calories they're actually consuming and may gain weight on their raw food diet. Oil has 4,000 calories per pound! A little bit goes a very long way, calorie-wise. As shown in table 9.1, nuts and seeds range from 2,500 to 2,750 calories per pound. Soaking nuts and seeds decreases their calorie density to about 1,800 calories per pound, which is still well above Dr. Rolls' guidelines for food choices that lead to optimum weight. However, nuts and seeds can still make a positive contribution to a raw diet, as long as plenty of vegetables are included at the same meal so the overall calorie density will average out to a more appropriate level. Sea vegetables, such as the dulse in table 9.1, have a high calorie density when dried, but sea vegetables are usually soaked in water first and usually eaten in relatively small portions, so their calorie contribution to the diet is typically low.

Water and fiber content play an important role in the calorie density of legumes and grains. Legumes and grains gain water when cooked and therefore become less calorie dense. The calorie density of unsoaked and unsprouted lentils is 1,601 calories per pound, in comparison to the calorie density of cooked lentils, which is 526 calories per pound. The values for uncooked whole grains versus cooked grains follow a similar pattern. For example, bread cooked in the oven, where it loses water, is more calorie dense than grains cooked in water, where they absorb water. High-fiber whole-grain bread is less calorie dense than low-fiber white bread.

The calorie density of meat and meat products varies depending on the fat and water content, as meat and meat products do not contain fiber. Cooked ham has a calorie density of 815 calories per pound, while the calorie density of fried bacon is 2,418 calories per pound. Bacon has more fat than ham and less water than ham when fried. Dairy products follow a similar pattern, since two-percent milk has a calorie density of 225 calories per pound, while the calorie density of American cheese is 1,500 calories per pound and butter is 3,275 calories per pound. Milk contains the most water and the least fat of these foods.

**Table 9.2.** The calorie densities of various legumes and legume sprouts

| Food | Calorie density (calories per pound) |
|------|--------------------------------------|
| Alfalfa sprouts | 104 |
| Alfalfa seeds | 873 |
| Lentil sprouts | 480 |
| Lentils, cooked | 526 |
| Lentils, unsoaked and unsprouted | 1,601 |
| Mung bean sprouts | 136 |
| Mung beans, unsoaked and unsprouted | 1,574 |
| Pea sprouts | 562 |
| Peas, dry, unsoaked and unsprouted | 1,547 |

During the cooking process lentils gain water, so their calorie density decreases to less than one-third of the original value. When soaked and sprouted, lentils decrease in calorie density to 480 calories per pound. Other legumes take on more water than lentils during soaking and sprouting. Mung bean sprouts and alfalfa sprouts are similar in calorie density to vegetables. Therefore, it would be next to impossible to get all one's calories from these low-calorie density sprouts.

**Table 9.3.** Calorie density of common sweeteners

| Food | Calorie density (calories per pound) |
|------|--------------------------------------|
| Blackstrap molasses | 1,080 |
| Maple syrup | 1,185 |
| Agave syrup | 1,296 |
| Honey | 1,380 |
| White sugar | 1,755 |

The sweeteners in table 9.3 have high calorie densities, so a little goes a long way. Keep in mind that most sweeteners are low in or devoid of important nutrients, so I encourage people to use whole-food sweeteners, such as dates or other fruit, as an alternative.

## Calorie Density in Practice

Here's an example of a salad and dressing that illustrates the difference in calorie density between vegetables and nuts or seeds.

---

### Garden Vegetable Salad

4 cups (188 g) chopped romaine lettuce
4 cups (99 g) chopped dandelion greens
1 cup (180 g) chopped tomatoes
1 cup (110 g) grated carrots
1 cup (104 g) chopped cucumber
1 cup (101 g) chopped celery
½ cup (21.2 g) chopped fresh basil

### Salad Dressing

2 cups (248 g) chopped zucchini
1 cup (149 g) chopped red bell pepper
½ cup (122 g) fresh-squeezed lemon juice
2 tablespoons (18 g) almonds
2 tablespoons (20 g) chia seeds
2 tablespoons (18 g) unhulled sesame seeds

---

**Table 9.4.** Macronutrients in large garden vegetable salad

|  | Vegetables and lemon juice | Nut and seeds | Total |
|---|---|---|---|
| Calories (kcal) | 307 | 304 | 611 |
| Carbohydrate (g) | 68.05 | 16.86 | 84.9 |
| Protein (g) | 14.57 | 10.11 | 24.7 |
| Fat (g) | 3.20 | 23.92 | 27.1 |

There are 611 calories in this salad and dressing, which is a little more than one-quarter of my calorie intake for one day, given that my calorie intake is usually around 2,000 calories per day and can be more or less depending on my activity level. The approximate percentages of calories from macronutrients in this salad and dressing are 45 percent from carbohydrate, 16 percent from protein, and 39 percent from fat. This example illustrates both the importance of water and fat content for determining calorie density. The higher the water content of a food, the lower the calorie density, and the higher the fat content, the higher the calorie density. The rest of my daily diet usually consists predominantly of fruit and greens, bringing the percentage of calories from fat for the whole day down considerably.

Imagine this large bowl of vegetables next to the small amount of nuts and seeds used to make the dressing. Even though the volume or weight of nuts and seeds in this recipe is small when compared to the vegetables, the calorie contribution from the nuts and seeds is similar to that of the vegetables. (See table 9.4 on the previous page.) Fat calories add up very quickly on a raw diet if fruit intake is restricted, given that the majority of calories on a raw plant-based diet are obtained from sweet fruits, nuts, seeds, avocados, coconuts, oils, calorie-containing sweeteners, and possibly sprouted dehy-

---

### Basic Green Smoothie
2 medium bananas (236 g)
3 cups (108 g) chopped collard greens
1 cup (237 ml) fresh-squeezed orange juice
½ cup (74 g) fresh blueberries
½ cup (62.5 g) fresh raspberries

Calories: 421 kcal, carbohydrate: 105.06 g, protein: 8 g, fat: 1.97 g
Approximate percentages of calories from macronutrients:
Carbohydrate: 88%, protein: 8%, fat: 4%

### Basic Almond Loaf
1 cup (110 g) grated carrots
1 cup (101 g) diced celery
¾ cup (107 g) soaked almonds
½ cup (80 g) chopped yellow onion
1 teaspoon (4.5 g) olive oil
1 teaspoon savory culinary herb of choice (optional, not included in nutrient analysis)

Calories: 749.7, carbohydrate: 44.25 g, protein: 25.36 g, fat: 58.02 g
Approximate percentages of calories from macronutrients:
Carbohydrate: 17%, protein: 14%, fat: 69%

---

drated grains. This doesn't imply that all fat is bad, given that some fats are essential and very important for health. It simply means that their contribution to calories shouldn't be overlooked, especially if achieving optimum weight is your goal.

For comparison purposes, see the two raw recipes on the facing page. One is a fruit-rich smoothie and the other is a fat-rich almond loaf. Once again, since fruits are naturally low in fat and high in carbohydrate, most of the calories in the smoothie come from the carbohydrates in the fruit. Even though vegetables constitute the majority of the almond loaf (2½ cups of vegetables out of the 3⅓ cups total), the largest calorie sources in this dish are almonds and olive oil. Fat contributes by far the most calories in the dish, 69 percent.

Once blended or mixed, the final volume of each of these recipes comes out to approximately 3 cups. Despite this, the fruit and green smoothie has just over half the amount of calories compared to the almond loaf. This is another real-world example of the types of dietary choices raw-food enthusiasts make, and how water, fat, and fiber have major influences over the amount of calories consumed.

## The Importance of Eating Enough
When people transition to a raw plant-based diet, they may not realize that the food they're now eating can be much less calorie dense than the food they were eating previously. On a standard Western diet, people tend to eat much smaller portions of more calorie-dense foods. When they shift their diet to focus on raw foods, they may not significantly increase their intake of vegetables. Often, I see new raw-food enthusiasts eating small dinner-sized salads and complain of being hungry after eating. This makes sense, because if someone is eating a raw diet structured around their previous diet but they eliminate cooked foods and animal foods and don't increase their intake of vegetables, they may be left feeling hungry.

For instance, instead of eating my very large garden salad (on page 123), they might eat a salad that's one-quarter that size. Not only will they get 25 percent of the calories, they'll only get 25 percent of all the nutrients as well. Table 9.5 on page 126 shows a sampling of the nutrients found in my large garden salad and dressing. For 611 calories, this nutrient profile is impressive. If one were to eat a salad one half or one quarter this size, they would adjust the nutrient content by dividing each nutrient by 2 and 4, respectively.

This 611-calorie salad illustrates the importance of eating vegetables in quantity for nutrient content and satiety. Raw fruits and vegetables are less calorie dense than many cooked foods, so it's important to be mindful of this when making a transition to eating more fruits and vegetables. Most people associate eating a greater volume of food with weight gain, but on a raw diet that focuses on fruits and vegetables, eating that increased volume is important in order to get enough essential nutrients, as well as calories. (See table 9.5.) At the same time, one has to be mindful of the more calorie-dense raw foods discussed earlier: nuts, seeds, avocados, coconut, oil, and sweeteners.

**Table 9.5.** Vitamins and minerals in the garden vegetable salad and dressing, p.123

|  | Salad and dressing | Adult DRI |
|---|---|---|
| A (RAE) | 2,659 | 700–900 |
| Beta-carotene (mcg) | 29,250 | NA |
| $B_1$ (mg) | 0.9 | 1.1–1.2 |
| $B_2$ (mg) | 1.3 | 1.1–1.3 |
| $B_3$ (mg) | 8.4 | 14–16 |
| $B_5$ (mg) | 2.5 | 5 |
| $B_6$ (mg) | 2 | 1.3–1.7 |
| Folate/$B_9$ (mcg) | 571.1 | 400 |
| $B_{12}$ (mcg) | 0 | 2.4 |
| C (mg) | 407.5 | 75–90 |
| D (IU) | 0 | 600–800 |
| E (mg) | 13.4 | 15 |
| Calcium (mg) | 801.1 | 1,000–1,200 |
| Copper (mcg) | 1,710 | 900 |
| Iron (mg) | 11.7 | 8–18 |
| Magnesium (mg) | 311.6 | 310–420 |
| Manganese (mg) | 3.3 | 1.8–2.3 |
| Potassium (mg) | 3,471.7 | 4,700 |
| Sodium (mg) | 296.9 | 1,200–1,500 |
| Zinc (mg) | 5.7 | 8–11 |

## Computing Calorie Needs

As we've seen, getting the right number of calories from a varied diet helps ensure adequate intake of macronutrients and micronutrients. If someone eats only 400 calories per day, they're not likely to get enough nutrients no matter how you combine them.

Most of us don't get out charts, graphs, and scales in order to determine our calorie intakes, but it's not a bad idea to have a sense of what's appropriate for your needs. A formula known as the Harris-Benedict equation is useful for determining approximately how many calories should be consumed daily to maintain weight based on body mass and activity level, among other factors. First, the basal metabolic rate (BMR) is calculated; this is the amount of calories needed to maintain weight without any activity taken into account. The formula is different for men and women:

United States customary units (pounds and inches):

For men, BMR = 66 + (6.26 x weight in lbs) + (12.7 x height in inches) – (6.8 x age in years)

For women, BMR = 655 + (4.35 x weight in lbs) + (4.7 x height in inches) – (4.7 x age in years)

International system of units (metric system):

For men, BMR = 66 + (13.7 x weight in kg) + (5 x height in cm) – (6.8 x age in years)

For women, BMR = 655 + (9.6 x weight in kg) + (1.8 x height in cm) – (4.7 x age in years)

To calculate the BMR calorie needs for a 40-year-old, 5-foot 10-inch, 150-pound male who is moderately active:

BMR = 66 + (6.26 x 150 = 939) + (12.7 x 70 = 889) – (6.8 x 40 = 272)

66 + 939 + 889 – 272 = 1,622 BMR

Everyone has a unique biochemical makeup, which includes their individual metabolic rate. But this formula provides a reasonable basis for calculating how many calories are needed.

Next, an activity factor is calculated into the equation. The more active someone is, the more calories they need to consume to maintain body weight. Multiplying the BMR times an activity factor (shown in table 9.6) results in the calories needed daily, or CND.

**Table 9.6.** The activity factor of various activity levels

| Activity level | Example | Activity factor |
|---|---|---|
| Little to no exercise | Sedentary, desk job | 1.2 |
| Light exercise | 1–3x/week | 1.375 |
| Moderate exercise | 3–5x/week | 1.55 |
| Heavy exercise | 6–7x/week | 1.75 |
| Very heavy exercise | 2x/day | 1.9 |

If the 150-pound man exercises moderately, his activity factor is 1.55. Multiplying that times his BMR of 1,622 results in a CND of 2,514 to maintain weight, approximately the 2,500 calories given in several of the sample menus and food analyses throughout the book. If this man is sedentary (not the best for optimal health!), then his activity factor is 1.2. CND is then the BMR of 1,622 x 1.2, which equals 1,946. Many sample menus and analyses throughout the book also contain approximately this number of calories.

The versions of the Harris-Benedict equation listed in this chapter are the ones most commonly used; however, the updated versions of the equation in the international system of units (metric system) are:

For men, BMR = 88.362 + (13.397 x weight in kg) + (4.799 x height in cm) – (5.677 x age in years)

For women, BMR = 447.593 + (9.247 x weight in kg) + (3.098 x height in cm) – (4.330 x age in years)

Using these versions of the equation gives very similar results to the more commonly used versions, but I provided the updates here for your reference.

## CHAPTER 10
# Nutrient Analyses of Various Raw Food Diets

—— ∞∞ ——

SINCE STARTING ON THIS PATH IN 1990, I've seen numerous trends come and go in the raw community, but the most persistent issue seems to be what's the best raw diet. Should it be one that includes more fruit or less fruit, how much fat is optimal, should someone eat 100 percent raw or include some cooked food, grains versus no grains, plant-based versus some animal foods, and what's the best way to get enough protein. I'm sure these debates will continue for some time, given the strong feelings, personal results, current personal health status, and beliefs held by people on all sides of the issues. Many of my students have expressed confusion about the seemingly opposing approaches to raw diets and which one is "right" or best.

Perhaps there are so many unique styles of raw-eating plans because different strategies work for different people, depending on their current circumstances, health situation and goals, bioindividuality, the way their body utilizes calories, or a variety of other reasons. On numerous occasions I have been surprised at people's expressed health outcomes, so I find myself maintaining an open mind about dietary choices. An evidence-based approach to diet is the most objective way to determine a course of action, and I prefer to let results or data speak for themselves.

Over the years, I've seen people employ many different approaches to raw food. Some have been successful short-term, but have changed their approach over time. Rarely have I observed someone start out with one particular approach and stick with it in that exact form. Most people modify their dietary choices as they become more experienced, become more tuned into the needs of their bodies, educate themselves about different approaches to raw or other dietary approaches, have lab testing done, talk to health care practitioners, start or modify exercise habits, experience a change in personal circumstances, or change their health focus.

There are as many types of raw food diets as there are people who eat them, but there are two main camps, which we refer to as the high-sweet fruit camp (high-fruit) and the low-sweet fruit camp (low-fruit). The menu plans that follow are examples of these diets, along with descriptions and tables of the nutrients they contain. The actual application of these approaches can be widely varied to suit the availability of produce and personal preferences.

### Daily Requirements for Macronutrients

The DRI for calories depends on a number of factors, including height, weight, age, sex, activity level, and other considerations, and is explained on pages 126–128. The DRIs for fat (20 to 35 percent of calories) have been challenged by some clinicians and health enthusiasts who would like to see that value lower than 20 percent—closer to or at 10 percent. Personal health status and athletic performance are two of the reasons often cited for choosing the low-fat dietary approach in high-sweet fruit raw diets. The protein RDA (10 to 15 percent of calories) is 46 grams for a woman and 56 grams for a man, but it's important to note that these numbers, as with calories, can vary depending upon someone's weight, activity level, and other factors, as explained on pages 30–32.

## High-Sweet Fruit Menu (2,000 kcal)

A high-sweet fruit menu plan may appear to have a lot of food, but consuming this much is not unusual for high-fruit raw-food enthusiasts. Fruit is much less calorie dense than nuts, seeds, grains, legumes, dehydrated foods, and heavier cooked foods, so one has to eat a larger amount of fruit to obtain enough calories to maintain weight and energy levels while not feeling hungry. Table 10.1 on the facing page shows the macronutrient content of the sample menu measured in grams and as a percentage of calories.

As shown in table 10.2 (page 132), the daily value has been met on this menu for vitamins $B_1$, $B_2$, $B_3$, $B_5$, $B_6$, C, and E and folate. Vitamins $B_{12}$ and D can be challenging to get on any diet, regardless of whether or not the diet contains animal products. The retinol activity equivalent of vitamin A for this menu is well beyond the daily value.

This high-sweet fruit menu provides more than the daily value for calcium for most adults, as well as iron, magnesium, potassium, and copper. This menu is a little short on zinc for men, as fruit is generally lower in zinc than nuts and seeds. For anyone who wants to add more zinc to their diet, wild rice, lentils, quinoa, leafy greens, sesame seeds, poppy seeds, and pumpkin seeds are good sources. This menu is also low in selenium, but Brazil nuts are a great source, given that one average-sized Brazil nut (4.75 g) contains 91 micrograms of selenium, which is about 165 percent of the daily value. Sweet fruits are a rich source of potassium and magnesium, which would account for the notable content of both in this menu.

The calcium content of this menu exceeds the daily value, but a large amount of the calcium is found in the spinach. As mentioned previously in the mineral chapter, it's preferable not to count on high-oxalate foods as a main source of calcium in a raw diet, but rather to focus on foods that are low in oxalate and high in calcium. This doesn't mean that spinach and other high-oxalate foods are not nutritious. They actually contain many other important nutrients besides calcium, such as beta-carotene and vitamin $K_1$. A number of lower-oxalate alternatives to spinach, such as kale, can be found on page 72. The reason I include spinach in this nutrient analysis is because I see many raw-food enthusiasts counting on spinach as their main leafy green. For this reason and others, I encourage the use of a variety of leafy greens.

This 2,000-calorie high-sweet fruit diet also provides more than the World Health Organization's recommendations for all the total protein and essential amino acids for anyone weighing between 120 and 150 pounds, as seen on pages 44–47. See table 10.3 (page 133) for amounts.

## High-Sweet Fruit Menu

### Breakfast
1 large cantaloupe (1,360 g)

### Lunch
4 medium bananas (472 g)
5 cups (227 g) chopped
    romaine lettuce
1½ cups (227 g) fresh
    blueberries

### Afternoon Snack
13 fresh apricots (454 g)
5 fresh figs (250 g)

### Dinner
Soup
3¾ cups (340 g) chopped broccoli
2 medium red bell peppers, chopped
    (227 g)
1¼ cup (227 g) chopped tomatoes
5 leaves fresh basil (2.5 g)

Salad
5 cups (227 g) chopped romaine lettuce
½ to ⅔ bunch baby spinach (227 g)
2¼ cups (227 g) diced celery

Salad Dressing
Mango, pit and skin removed (207 g)
Juice of 1 lemon (3 oz/84 g)
1 tablespoon (15 g) sesame tahini

**Table 10.1.** Macronutrients in the sample high-sweet fruit raw menu

| Nutrient | Amount in menu | Percentage of calories |
|---|---|---|
| Calories | 2,051 | - |
| Carbohydrate | 466.7 g | 80 |
| Protein | 58.3 g | 11 |
| Fat | 19.7 g | 9 |
| Saturated fat | 3.2 g | - |
| Water content | 4,181 ml | - |

**Table 10.2.** Vitamins and minerals in the sample high-sweet fruit raw menu

| Nutrient | Amount in menu | Adult DRI |
|---|---|---|
| **Vitamins** | | |
| A (RAE) | 6,508 | 700–900 |
| Beta-carotene (mcg) | 76,649 | - |
| B₁ (mg) | 2.3 | 1.1–1.2 |
| B₂ (mg) | 2.6 | 1.1–1.3 |
| B₃ (mg) | 28.4 | 14–16 |
| B₅ (mg) | 9.1 | 5 |
| B₆ (mg) | 5.8 | 1.3–1.7 |
| Folate/B₉ (mcg) | 1,977 | 400 |
| B₁₂ (mcg) | 0 | 2.4 |
| C (mg) | 1,516 | 75–90 |
| D (IU) | 0 | 600–800 |
| E (mg) | 22.2 | 15 |
| **Minerals** | | |
| Calcium (mg) | 1,091 | 1,000–1,200 |
| Copper (mcg) | 2,840 | 900 |
| Iron (mg) | 23.3 | 8–18 |
| Magnesium (mg) | 777 | 310–420 |
| Manganese (mg) | 7.4 | 1.8–2.3 |
| Potassium (mg) | 12,181 | 4,700 |
| Selenium (mcg) | 26 | 55 |
| Sodium (mg) | 776 | 1,200–1,500 |
| Zinc (mg) | 10.1 | 8–11 |

Many people who eat a high-sweet fruit raw diet are very physically active and must eat more calories when working out or training than when sedentary to support their energy needs. The addition of eight bananas and two figs to the 2,000-calorie high-fruit menu would bring the calorie level up to 3,000. Naturally, this addition would also contribute more carbohydrate, protein, fat, phytonutrients, antioxidants, vitamins, and minerals than the basic menu (see table 10.4), because the whole-food content increased. The percentage of calories from each macronutrient, however, is slightly different from the basic 2,000-calorie high-sweet fruit menu. The reason why the percentage of calories from protein decreased from the basic menu is because the foods that were added were fruits, which have comparatively more carbohydrate and less protein than vegetables. Despite this change, the total amount of protein (71.14 grams) well exceeds the average daily values of 46 grams for women and 56 grams for men.

**Table 10.3.** Amino acid content in the sample high-sweet fruit menu

| Amino acid (g) | Amount in menu | WHO recommendations g/54 kg (120 lbs) | WHO recommendations g/68 kg (150 lbs) |
|---|---|---|---|
| Histidine | 1.33 | 0.54 | 0.68 |
| Isoleucine | 1.73 | 1.09 | 1.36 |
| Leucine | 2.90 | 2.14 | 2.65 |
| Lysine | 2.61 | 1.63 | 2.04 |
| Methionine (+ cysteine) | 1.12 | 0.82 | 1.02 |
| Phenylalanine (+ tyrosine) | 3.39 | 1.36 | 1.70 |
| Threonine | 1.72 | 0.82 | 1.02 |
| Tryptophan | 0.52 | 0.22 | 0.27 |
| Valine | 2.35 | 1.42 | 1.77 |

**Table 10.4.** Macronutrients in the 3,000-calorie high-fruit raw menu

| Nutrient | Amount in menu | Percentage of calories |
|---|---|---|
| Calories | 3,012 | - |
| Carbohydrate | 695.9 g | 82 |
| Protein | 71.1 g | 9 |
| Fat | 28.9 g | 9 |
| Saturated fat | 5.1 g | - |
| Water content | 4,943 ml | - |

## Low-Sweet Fruit Menu

On the other end of the raw-food spectrum is the low-sweet fruit approach. Many low-sweet fruit menus contain large amounts of sprouts, for which there is little nutrient information in nutrition databases, so I look forward to a time when this information is available. Although not all low-sweet fruit raw foodists eat large quantities of vegetables, this nutrient analysis reflects a high vegetable approach to a low-sweet fruit raw diet.

The only sweet fruit on this menu is the banana, and menus representative of this approach may have this amount of fruit or even less. Vegetables, including leafy greens and sprouts, don't contain a significant number of calories. Vegetables, on average, are about 100 calories per pound, and it would be difficult, if not impossible, to eat the amount of vegetables, greens, and/or sprouts necessary to get enough calories.

Calories have to come from somewhere, and most of the calories on 100-percent raw and low-sweet fruit diets end up coming from fat. Many people who eat this way don't realize the amount of fat they're consuming as a percentage of calories. As was discussed on page 119, when fat is reported by weight or volume, the fat content of these menu plans may appear smaller than it is because of the water and fiber content of the foods in the plans. Calculating this as a percentage of calories, as is done in table 10.5 (page 136), more accurately reveals the true fat content.

The protein content is higher on the low-sweet fruit menu than the high-sweet fruit menu, because vegetables in general have more protein than fruit and sweet fruits have comparatively more carbohydrate than vegetables. Like the high-sweet fruit menu, this low-sweet fruit menu has more than the daily value for vitamins $B_1$, $B_2$, $B_3$, $B_5$, $B_6$, C, and E and folate and has a notable amount of beta-carotene.

As on the high-sweet fruit menu, the iron, magnesium, potassium, copper, and manganese levels are excellent. Calcium content is also excellent and is greater than that of the 2,000-calorie high-sweet fruit menu, as is the content of magnesium and zinc. Potassium content is smaller than that of the high-sweet fruit menu but is still excellent. Fruit is a richer source of potassium than vegetables and fat sources. Once again, Brazil nuts are a great source of selenium and can easily help to meet the daily value.

This menu plan has the lowest sodium so far, likely because the high-sweet fruit plan contains celery, which is naturally rich in sodium. A whole-foods, plant-based raw diet with no added salt or products containing added salt, generally contains 300 to 500 milligrams of sodium, depending on whether or not the menu contains sodium-rich foods, such as celery or sea vegetables. The sodium content of this menu can be increased by adding celery or another sodium-rich food.

The amino acid content of this menu plan exceeds the daily value for total protein and every essential amino acid for individuals who weigh between 120 and 150 pounds, also as seen on pages 47–50. When compared to the high-sweet fruit menu, the essential amino acid content in this menu is greater, with the exception of lysine.

The low-sweet fruit menu includes more vegetables, nuts, seeds, and avocados than the high-sweet fruit menu. This doesn't imply that all high-sweet fruit menus are lower in vegetables than the menu on the facing page. Some high-sweet fruit enthusiasts wisely include large amounts of vegetables in their diet, so the vegetable content of a diet can certainly vary with each individual approach.

## Low-Sweet Fruit Menu

### Breakfast
Blended Quinoa Cereal
½ cup (85 g) dry quinoa, sprouted (approximate yield: 1 cup)
½ cup (237 ml) water
½ ripe banana (59 g)
½ teaspoon (1.3 g) cinnamon
½ cup (71.5 g) unsoaked almonds, for garnish

### Lunch
Sprouted Lentil and Vegetable Soup
2 cups (202 g) chopped celery
1 cup (180 g) chopped tomatoes
⅓ cup (64 g) dry lentils, sprouted (approximate yield: 1⅓ cups)
½ medium avocado (68 g)
1 green onion (25 g)

### Dinner
Salad
4 cups (188 g) chopped romaine lettuce
4 cups (99 g) chopped dandelion greens
1 cup (180 g) chopped tomatoes
1 cup (110 g) grated carrots
1 cup (104 g) chopped cucumber
½ cup (21.2 g) chopped fresh basil

Salad Dressing
2 cups (298 g) chopped red bell pepper
2 cups (248 g) chopped zucchini
½ cup (122 g) fresh-squeezed lemon juice
2 tablespoons (18 g) almonds
2 tablespoons (20 g) chia seeds
2 tablespoons (18 g) unhulled sesame seeds

### Evening Snack
¼ cup (36 g) almonds

**Table 10.5.** Macronutrients in the 2,000-calorie low-sweet fruit raw menu

| Nutrient | Amount in menu | Percentage of calories |
|---|---|---|
| Calories | 2,038 | - |
| Carbohydrate | 242.4 g | 41 |
| Protein | 82.2 g | 16 |
| Fat | 97.7 g | 43 |
| Saturated fat | 9.5 g | - |
| Water content | 1,773 ml | - |

**Table 10.6.** Vitamins and minerals in the sample low-sweet fruit raw menu

| Nutrient | Amount in menu | Adult DRI |
|---|---|---|
| **Vitamins** | | |
| A (RAE) | 3,011 | 700–900 |
| Beta-carotene (mcg) | 32,982 | - |
| $B_1$ (mg) | 2.3 | 1.1–1.2 |
| $B_2$ (mg) | 3.2 | 1.1–1.3 |
| $B_3$ (mg) | 19.6 | 14–16 |
| $B_5$ (mg) | 7.1 | 5 |
| $B_6$ (mg) | 4 | 1.3–1.7 |
| Folate/$B_9$ (mcg) | 1,308 | 400 |
| $B_{12}$ (mcg) | 0 | 2.4 |
| C (mg) | 642 | 75–90 |
| D (IU) | 0 | 600–800 |
| E (mg) | 49 | 15 |
| **Minerals** | | |
| Calcium (mg) | 1,272 | 1,000–1,200 |
| Copper (mcg) | 3,970 | 900 |
| Iron (mg) | 26.8 | 8–18 |
| Magnesium (mg) | 934.8 | 310–420 |
| Manganese (mg) | 9.4 | 1.8–2.3 |
| Potassium (mg) | 6,952 | 4,700 |
| Selenium (mcg) | 21.2 | 55 |
| Sodium (mg) | 412 | 1,200–1,500 |
| Zinc (mg) | 16.2 | 8–11 |

**Table 10.7.** Amino acid content in the sample low-sweet fruit menu

| Amino acid (g) | Amount in menu | WHO recommendations g/54 kg (120 lbs) | WHO recommendations g/68 kg (150 lbs) |
|---|---|---|---|
| Histidine | 1.51 | 0.54 | 0.68 |
| Isoleucine | 2.01 | 1.09 | 1.36 |
| Leucine | 3.71 | 2.14 | 2.65 |
| Lysine | 2.36 | 1.63 | 2.04 |
| Methionine (+ cysteine) | 1.46 | 0.82 | 1.02 |
| Phenylalanine (+ tyrosine) | 4.31 | 1.36 | 1.70 |
| Threonine | 1.92 | 0.82 | 1.02 |
| Tryptophan | 0.74 | 0.22 | 0.27 |
| Valine | 2.43 | 1.42 | 1.77 |

## Intermediate Raw Menu

Most of the raw-food enthusiasts that I've met over the years eat somewhere in between a high-sweet fruit and low-sweet fruit diet. I've also found that most people who stick to a primarily raw diet long-term have an approach that is somewhere in between these two plans; Dr. Rick and I do as well.

When compared to the 2,000-calorie high-sweet fruit and low-sweet fruit menus, the menu plan on page 138 is intermediate in terms of carbohydrate, protein, and fat content. The protein content of this menu plan meets or exceeds the daily value for total protein and every essential amino acid for individuals who weigh between 120 and 150 pounds. It's superior to the low-sweet fruit menu in vitamins $B_3$, $B_5$, $B_6$, C and beta-carotene. It's also equivalent to the 2,000-calorie high-sweet fruit menu in vitamins $B_1$, $B_2$, and $B_6$. Overall this menu exceeds the daily value for the vitamins listed in table 10.8 (page 139), with the exception of vitamins $B_{12}$ and D, which can be challenging to acquire regardless of one's diet.

This menu plan also exceeds the daily value in all the minerals listed in table 10.8, with the exception of sodium. Sodium content is higher than in the low-sweet fruit menu, likely because of the celery content. Calcium is the highest of any of the menus so far. The potassium, sodium, and manganese content falls between that of the high-sweet fruit and low-sweet fruit menus, and selenium exceeds the daily value due to the inclusion of a Brazil nut. Please note that the soup recipe in this menu is slightly different from the one in the low-sweet fruit menu, as it contains fewer sprouted lentils.

## Intermediate Raw Menu

### Breakfast
Green Smoothie
4 medium bananas (472 g)
2 medium oranges (242 g)
3 cups (201 g) chopped kale
2 cups (330 g) sliced mango
1 cup (148 g) fresh blueberries

### Morning Snack
5 fresh figs (250 g)

### Lunch
Green Soup
2 cups (202 g) chopped celery
1 cup (180 g) chopped tomatoes
½ medium avocado (68 g)
⅓ cup (39 g) sprouted lentils
1 green onion (25 g)

### Afternoon Snack
5 fresh figs (250 g)

### Dinner
Salad
8 cups (376 g) chopped romaine lettuce
4 cups (99 g) chopped dandelion greens
1 cup (180 g) chopped tomatoes
1 cup (110 g) grated carrots
1 cup (104 g) chopped cucumber
½ cup (21.2 g) chopped fresh basil

Salad Dressing
1 cup (149 g) chopped red bell pepper
1 cup (124 g) chopped zucchini
¼ cup (61 g) fresh-squeezed lemon juice
2 tablespoons (20 g) chia seeds
1 tablespoon (9 g) almonds
1 tablespoon (9 g) unhulled sesame seeds

### Evening Snack
1 Brazil nut (4.73 g)

**Table 10.7.** Macronutrients in the sample intermediate raw menu

| Nutrient | Amount in menu | Percentage of calories |
|----------|----------------|------------------------|
| Calories | 2,039 | - |
| Carbohydrate | 431.2 g | 71 |
| Protein | 61.8 g | 12 |
| Fat | 39.5 g | 17 |
| Saturated fat | 5.81 g | - |
| Water content | 3,110 ml | - |

**Table 10.8.** Vitamins and minerals in the sample intermediate raw menu

| Nutrient | Amount in menu | Adult DRI |
|----------|----------------|-----------|
| **Vitamins** | | |
| A (RAE) | 5,334 | 700–900 |
| Beta-carotene (mcg) | 60,804 | - |
| $B_1$ (mg) | 2.3 | 1.1–1.2 |
| $B_2$ (mg) | 2.6 | 1.1–1.3 |
| $B_3$ (mg) | 21 | 14–16 |
| $B_5$ (mg) | 8.6 | 5 |
| $B_6$ (mg) | 5.8 | 1.3–1.7 |
| Folate/$B_9$ (mcg) | 1,264 | 400 |
| $B_{12}$ (mcg) | 0 | 2.4 |
| C (mg) | 959 | 75–90 |
| D (IU) | 0 | 600–800 |
| E (mg) | 20 | 15 |
| **Minerals** | | |
| Calcium (mg) | 1,436 | 1,000–1,200 |
| Copper (mcg) | 3,550 | 900 |
| Iron (mg) | 21.3 | 8–18 |
| Magnesium (mg) | 683 | 310–420 |
| Manganese (mg) | 7.7 | 1.8–2.3 |
| Potassium (mg) | 9,450 | 4,700 |
| Selenium (mcg) | 105 | 55 |
| Sodium (mg) | 504 | 1,200–1,500 |
| Zinc (mg) | 9.2 | 8–11 |

**Table 10.9.** Amino acid content in the sample intermediate raw menu

| Amino acid (g) | Amount in menu | WHO recommendations g/54 kg (120 lbs) | WHO recommendations g/68 kg (150 lbs) |
|---|---|---|---|
| Histidine | 1.16 | 0.54 | 0.68 |
| Isoleucine | 1.58 | 1.09 | 1.36 |
| Leucine | 2.68 | 2.14 | 2.65 |
| Lysine | 2.14 | 1.63 | 2.04 |
| Methionine (+ cysteine) | 1.11 | 0.82 | 1.02 |
| Phenylalanine (+ tyrosine) | 3.15 | 1.36 | 1.70 |
| Threonine | 1.53 | 0.82 | 1.02 |
| Tryptophan | 0.52 | 0.22 | 0.27 |
| Valine | 1.94 | 1.42 | 1.77 |

# 80-Percent Raw Menu (20-Percent Cooked)

Some people choose to add some cooked whole foods to a primarily raw diet. The following example contains 80 percent of the calories from raw food and 20 percent from cooked foods. Steamed lentils and amaranth collectively contribute 350 calories, close to 20 percent of the total calories on this menu.

This menu exceeds the daily value for all the minerals listed in table 10.11 (page 142), with the exception of sodium, which can be increased by the addition of a sodium-rich food, such as celery or a small amount of some type of sea vegetable. With the exception of vitamins $B_{12}$ and D, this menu exceeds the daily value for the vitamins in table 10.11. The amino acid content of this menu plan exceeds the daily value for total protein and every essential amino acid for individuals who weigh between 120 and 150 pounds.

**Table 10.10.** Macronutrients in the sample 80-percent raw menu

| Nutrient | Amount in menu | Percentage of calories |
|---|---|---|
| Calories | 2,031 | - |
| Carbohydrate | 405.2 g | 70 |
| Protein | 62.3 g | 12 |
| Fat | 40.2 g | 18 |
| Saturated fat | 5.5 g | - |
| Water content | 2,532 ml | - |

### Breakfast
Green Smoothie
4 medium bananas (472 g)
3 cups (201 g) chopped kale
2 cups (330 g) sliced mango
2 medium oranges (242 g)
1 cup (148 g) fresh blueberries

### Morning Snack
3 fresh figs (150 g)

### Lunch
Steamed Lentils and Amaranth with Avocado
½ medium avocado (68 g)
⅓ cup (64 g) dry lentils, steamed
¼ cup (48 g) dry amaranth, steamed

### Dinner
Salad
8 cups (376 g) chopped romaine lettuce
4 cups (99 g) chopped dandelion greens
1 cup (180 g) chopped tomatoes
1 cup (110 g) grated carrots
1 cup (104 g) chopped cucumber
½ cup (21.2 g) chopped fresh basil

Salad Dressing
1 cup (149 g) chopped red bell pepper
1 cup (124 g) chopped zucchini
¼ cup (61 g) fresh-squeezed lemon juice
2 tablespoons (20 g) chia seeds
1 tablespoon (9 g) almonds
1 tablespoon (9 g) unhulled sesame seeds

### Evening Snack
1 Brazil nut (4.73 g)

**Table 10.11.** Vitamins and minerals in the sample 80-percent raw menu

| Nutrient | Amount in menu | Adult DRI |
|---|---|---|
| **Vitamins** | | |
| A (RAE) | 5,177 | 700–900 |
| Beta-carotene (mcg) | 59,019 | - |
| B₁ (mg) | 2.5 | 1.1–1.2 |
| B₂ (mg) | 2.4 | 1.1–1.3 |
| B₃ (mg) | 20 | 14–16 |
| B₅ (mg) | 8.1 | 5 |
| B₆ (mg) | 5.5 | 1.3–1.7 |
| Folate/B₉ (mcg) | 1,437 | 400 |
| B₁₂ (mcg) | 0 | 2.4 |
| C (mg) | 918 | 75–90 |
| D (IU) | 0 | 600–800 |
| E (mg) | 18 | 15 |
| **Minerals** | | |
| Calcium (mg) | 1,285 | 1,000–1,200 |
| Copper (mcg) | 3,530 | 900 |
| Iron (mg) | 25.4 | 8–18 |
| Magnesium (mg) | 726 | 310–420 |
| Manganese (mg) | 8.6 | 1.8–2.3 |
| Potassium (mg) | 8,314 | 4,700 |
| Selenium (mcg) | 116 | 55 |
| Sodium (mg) | 335 | 1,200–1,500 |
| Zinc (mg) | 11.7 | 8–11 |

**Table 10.12.** Amino acid content in the sample 80-percent raw menu

| Amino acid (g) | Amount in menu | WHO recommendations g/54 kg (120 lbs) | WHO recommendations g/68 kg (150 lbs) |
|---|---|---|---|
| Histidine | 1.24 | 0.54 | 0.68 |
| Isoleucine | 1.70 | 1.09 | 1.36 |
| Leucine | 2.69 | 2.14 | 2.65 |
| Lysine | 2.22 | 1.63 | 2.04 |
| Methionine (+ cysteine) | 1.14 | 0.82 | 1.02 |
| Phenylalanine (+ tyrosine) | 3.18 | 1.36 | 1.70 |
| Threonine | 1.62 | 0.82 | 1.02 |
| Tryptophan | 0.57 | 0.22 | 0.27 |
| Valine | 2.42 | 1.42 | 1.77 |

There are also other raw-food approaches, which include the gourmet raw approach and the use of superfoods and other products, such as algae, green-food powders, and goji berries. Many of the popular so-called super-foods and products popular in the raw community today are challenging to find in nutrient analysis programs, making it difficult to include them in nutrient analyses. For this reason and others, these products are not included in any of these menu plans.

## Standard Western Menu

For comparison purposes, I include a sample standard Western menu on page 144. Note that some eating patterns will include much more processed and fast food than is indicated here. Cooked foods and animal foods are generally much more calorie dense than fruits and vegetables, which is why there is comparatively less food and more calories on this menu versus the 2,000-calorie unprocessed plant-based menus in this chapter. Saturated fat content is the greatest of all the menus, and this is the first menu plan that contains cholesterol, a result of the animal food content. The daily values for vitamin $B_5$, vitamin $B_6$, folate, vitamin D, vitamin E, and vitamin A (RAE) were not met on this menu. Beta-carotene content is much smaller than the other menus, because the fruit and vegetable content is low. The daily values for calcium, iron, magnesium, potassium, zinc, copper, and manganese were not met with this menu, and sodium exceeds the upper limit of 2,300 milligrams.

I often hear criticism of vegan diets for not meeting vitamin D requirements, but more often than not I see menu plans based on animal products that are just as low in vitamin D. (See table 10.14 on page 145.) Vitamin D insufficiency and deficiency are widespread among the US population, of which the very large majority is not following a vegetarian, vegan, or raw food diet.

## Essential Fats in Various Menus

Plant-based diets are often under scrutiny because they don't contain traditional sources of omega-3 fats, such as cold-water fish. Given this, how do the sample raw diets hold up as far as the quantity of omega-3 fats and the ratio to omega-6 fats?

Table 10.16 (page 146) hows that all four of the raw food menus have favorable omega-6 to omega-3 ratios, and the amounts of ALA, the omega-3 essential (or parent) fat, on these menus are good. This is not surprising, based on the popular raw foods listed in table 3.1 (page 24).

Also not surprising, the omega-3 content of the standard Western diet is low, given that it doesn't contain significant amounts of cold-water fish,

## Standard Western Menu

### Breakfast
1 plain 4-inch bagel (105 g)
1 pat (1 inch x ⅓ inch) butter (5 g)
1 cup (237 ml) coffee

### Lunch
Ham and cheese sandwich with lettuce and tomato (146 g)
4-ounce bag (114 g) salted potato chips
12-ounce can (355 ml) diet soda

### Dinner
Entrée
4 ounces (113 g) roast beef
1 cup (210 g) mashed potatoes, with margarine and milk
1 cup (182 g) cooked frozen mixed vegetables

Salad
3 cups (414 g) tossed salad with iceberg lettuce, tomato, onion
1 tablespoon (15.6 g) thousand island dressing
8-ounce glass (244 ml) milk, 2% fat

**Table 10.13.** Macronutrients in the sample standard Western menu

| Nutrient | Amount in menu | Percentage of calories |
|---|---|---|
| Calories | 2,193 | - |
| Carbohydrate | 238.7 g | 42 |
| Protein | 93 g | 17 |
| Fat | 100 g | 41 |
| Saturated fat | 30 g | - |
| Water content | 1,329 ml | - |

**Table 10.14.** Vitamins and minerals in the sample standard Western menu

| Nutrient | Amount in menu | Adult DRI |
|---|---|---|
| **Vitamins** | | |
| A (RAE) | 663 | 700–900 |
| Beta-carotene (mcg) | 30 | - |
| B₁ (mg) | 1.6 | 1.1–1.2 |
| B₂ (mg) | 1.8 | 1.1–1.3 |
| B₃ (mg) | 19.3 | 14–16 |
| B₅ (mg) | 3.8 | 5 |
| B₆ (mg) | 1.4 | 1.3–1.7 |
| Folate/B₉ (mcg) | 397.5 | 400 |
| B₁₂ (mcg) | 4.1 | 2.4 |
| C (mg) | 134 | 75–90 |
| D (IU) | 108 | 600–800 |
| E (mg) | 1.4 | 15 |
| **Minerals** | | |
| Calcium (mg) | 546 | 1,000–1,200 |
| Copper (mcg) | 710 | 900 |
| Iron (mg) | 14.2 | 8–18 |
| Magnesium (mg) | 219 | 310–420 |
| Manganese (mg) | 1.4 | 1.8–2.3 |
| Potassium (mg) | 2,358 | 4,700 |
| Selenium (mcg) | 60 | 55 |
| Sodium (mg) | 3,259 | 1,200–1,500 |
| Zinc (mg) | 9.3 | 8–11 |

**Table 10.15.** Amino acid content in the sample standard Western menu

| Amino acid (g) | Amount in menu | WHO recommendations g/54 kg (120 lbs) | WHO recommendations g/68 kg (150 lbs) |
|---|---|---|---|
| Histidine | 2.26 | 0.54 | 0.68 |
| Isoleucine | 3.41 | 1.09 | 1.36 |
| Leucine | 5.91 | 2.14 | 2.65 |
| Lysine | 5.21 | 1.63 | 2.04 |
| Methionine (+ cysteine) | 2.86 | 0.82 | 1.02 |
| Phenylalanine (+ tyrosine) | 5.93 | 1.36 | 1.70 |
| Threonine | 2.84 | 0.82 | 1.02 |
| Tryptophan | 0.88 | 0.22 | 0.27 |
| Valine | 3.79 | 1.42 | 1.77 |

chia seeds, flaxseeds, or a significant amount of leafy greens. As mentioned on page 23, the omega-6 to omega-3 ratios of standard Western menus can fall in the range of 15:1 to 25:1. Standard Western menus that contain cold-water fish or fish oil supplements have more omega-3 in the form of DHA and EPA, but often in these cases the ratio is only slightly improved because of the generally high omega-6 content of this type of diet. This standard western menu contains no DHA. I've found that adding more fruits and vegetables and removing processed foods and other omega-6 sources can have a pro-found effect on the improvement of this ratio, depending on what changes are made and the degree to which changes are made.

**Table 10.16.** The omega fat content of sample menus

| Menu | omega-6 (%) | omega-3 (%) | omega-6:3 ratio | ALA (g) |
| --- | --- | --- | --- | --- |
| High-sweet fruit | 27 | 10 | 2.6:1 | 2 |
| Low-sweet fruit | 26 | 5 | 5.5:1 | 4.6 |
| Intermediate raw | 24 | 11 | 2.3:1 | 5.1 |
| 80-percent raw | 30 | 12 | 2.3:1 | 5 |
| Standard Western | 5 | 0.6 | 8:1 | 0.7 |

## The Final Analysis

The standard Western diet has been established for so long that it can be dif-ficult for some people to imagine anyone getting the proper nutrients without eating meat, fish, dairy, and grains and grain products. However, as these raw menus show, perhaps it's the standard Western diet that's lacking! The revealing evidence presented in this chapter will hopefully inspire anyone in doubt to reconsider their own diet.

## CHAPTER 11

# The Importance of Focusing on Whole Plant Foods

PEOPLE OFTEN ASK ME WHAT I THINK is the most important dietary consideration. The answer is easy—whole foods, foods in their natural state, as grown. I've seen people improve their health tremendously just by removing commercially processed or packaged foods from their diets and focusing on whole foods, both cooked and raw. I define commercially processed foods as those that may have had the water and fiber removed and sugar, salt, and/or fat added back in, along with a variety of additives.

Not everyone is ready to make the jump directly from the standard Western diet to a raw, plant-based diet, and often change to this extent may not even be necessary to improve health. There are steps that can be taken in between. Some people do better taking a gradual approach, while others are comfortable taking the complete plunge. I'm in favor of making small, incremental changes to allow some time to adjust and incorporate them into my daily routine. Rapid, far-reaching dietary changes can be a challenge for many people, which may lead to backsliding or pendulum eating, including a return to processed foods.

There are multiple, synergistic changes that can be made simultaneously when moving from a standard Western diet to a whole-foods, plant-based raw diet. When making this shift, a person may:

- Minimize or eliminate processed foods and emphasize whole foods.
- Increase fruits and vegetables, which may have been minimal in the previous diet. Some people significantly increase the leafy green content of their diet.
- Decrease animal products, eliminate them altogether, or switch over to locally grown or grass-fed sources.
- Reduce or eliminate cooked foods, or change the type of cooking methods used, such as moving from frying to steaming.
- Change the source of water, such as moving from municipal tap water to spring water or purified water.
- Decrease or eliminate gluten-containing foods and processed carbohydrates.

Making big changes at once can be a challenge. But if someone's having trouble maintaining a totally raw diet, eating just whole plant foods can be a part of a fallback plan that's still very healthful. Instead of backsliding to the standard Western diet, one can backslide to steamed vegetables. Instead of eating fast-food French fries, they can have a steamed yam. Cooked wild rice and lentils can replace bread. I happen to think that 100-percent raw may not be the best approach for everyone all the time. It's important to find the balance that works for someone's personal and health circumstances. Some people may experience fewer cravings if they make changes slowly. Others may find that the opposite is true.

In addition, whole foods contain nutrients that haven't been altered by processing. The vitamins, minerals, phytonutrients, fiber, water, carbohydrate, protein, and fat are present in this whole-food matrix and can work together synergistically. The nutrients, fiber, and water are often extracted from processed foods, only to be partially added back later in the form of chemical substitutes.

To be fair, not all processing methods are created equal. For example, cold pressing oil, which is the technique used to obtain olive oil, is different from other oil extraction methods. Nonetheless, olives are very different nutritionally than olive oil, and the same is true for coconuts and coconut oil. It's important to note that oils, at 4,000 calories per pound, are extremely calorie dense, and if you're eating a fair amount of oil on a daily basis, those calories add up quickly. In addition, all the calories in oils come without fiber, water, or protein and only a fraction of the vitamins, minerals, phytonutrients, and antioxidants found in the whole food. Although a little oil in someone's diet won't necessarily ruin their health, raw-food enthusiasts who use large amounts of oil in their recipes, on their salads, and in their smoothies will be missing out on almost all the nutrients found in whole-food sources—but none of the calories!

To illustrate this point, table 11.1 shows a nutrient comparison between coconut oil and coconut meat. The analysis is for mature coconut meat, given that the nutrient content of young coconut was not available. The calorie content of these two samples is almost identical, but there's quite a difference in all the nutrients, except fat.

Coconut meat is not exactly a nutrient powerhouse. It would take about 17 servings of 33 grams each to supply about 2,000 calories from coconut meat. If someone ate that much coconut meat in a day, they would meet their calorie needs but would be severely lacking in every single vitamin, mineral, and essential fatty acid listed in table 11.1. They would also be quite low in total protein and every single essential amino acid, as well as very low in fiber.

**Table 11.1.** A comparison of the nutrients in coconut oil and coconut meat

| Nutrient | Coconut oil (1 Tbsp/13.6 g) | Mature coconut meat (33 g) |
|---|---|---|
| Calories (kcal) | 117.2 | 116.8 |
| Carbohydrate (g) | 0 | 5 |
| Protein (g) | 0 | 1.1 |
| Fat (g) | 13.6 | 11.1 |
| Percentage of calories from fat | 100 | 86 |
| Saturated fat (g) | 11.8 | 9.8 |
| Monounsaturated fat (g) | 0.8 | 0.5 |
| Polyunsaturated fat (g) | 0.2 | 0.1 |

| **Vitamins** | | | Adult DRI |
|---|---|---|---|
| A (RAE) | 0 | 0 | 700–900 |
| Beta-carotene (mcg) | 0 | 0 | - |
| $B_1$ (mg) | 0 | 0.02 | 1.1–1.2 |
| $B_2$ (mg) | 0 | 0.01 | 1.1–1.3 |
| $B_3$ (mg) | 0 | 0.18 | 14–16 |
| $B_5$ (mg) | 0 | 0.10 | 5 |
| $B_6$ (mg) | 0 | 0.02 | 1.3–1.7 |
| Folate/$B_9$ (mcg) | 0 | 8.58 | 400 |
| $B_{12}$ (mcg) | 0 | 0 | 2.4 |
| C (mg) | 0 | 1.09 | 75–90 |
| D (IU) | 0 | 0 | 600–800 |
| E (mg) | 0.01 | 0.08 | 15 |
| **Minerals** | | | |
| Calcium (mg) | 0 | 4.62 | 1,000–1,200 |
| Copper (mcg) | 0 | 0.14 | 900 |
| Iron (mg) | 0.01 | 0.80 | 8–18 |
| Magnesium (mg) | 0 | 10.56 | 310–420 |
| Manganese (mg) | 0 | 0.50 | 1.8–2.3 |
| Potassium (mg) | 0 | 117.48 | 4,700 |
| Selenium (mcg) | 0 | 3.33 | 55 |
| Sodium (mg) | 0 | 6.60 | 1,200–1,500 |
| Zinc (mg) | 0 | 0.36 | 8–11 |

| Amino acids | Coconut oil (1 Tbsp/13.6 g) | Mature coconut meat (33 g) |
|---|---|---|
| Histidine (g) | 0 | 0.02 |
| Isoleucine (g) | 0 | 0.04 |
| Leucine (g) | 0 | 0.07 |
| Lysine (g) | 0 | 0.04 |
| Methionine (+ cysteine) (g) | 0 | 0.04 |
| Phenylalanine (+ tyrosine) (g) | 0 | 0.08 |
| Threonine (g) | 0 | 0.04 |
| Tryptophan (g) | 0 | 0.01 |
| Valine (g) | 0 | 0.06 |
| **Saturated fatty acids** | | |
| Butyric acid (g) | 0 | 0 |
| Caproic acid (g) | 0.08 | 0.06 |
| Caprylic acid (g) | 1.02 | 0.77 |
| Capric acid (g) | 0.82 | 0.62 |
| Lauric acid (g) | 6.07 | 4.90 |
| Myristic acid (g) | 2.28 | 1.94 |
| Pentadecylic acid (g) | 0 | 0 |
| Palmitic acid (g) | 1.12 | 0.94 |
| Stearic acid (g) | 0.38 | 0.57 |
| **Polyunsaturated fatty acids** | | |
| Linoleic acid (LA) omega-6 (g) | 0.24 | 0.12 |
| Alpha-linolenic acid (ALA) omega-3 (g) | 0 | 0 |
| Eicosapentaenoic acid (EPA) omega-3 (g) | 0 | 0 |
| Docosahexaenoic acid (DHA) omega-3 (g) | 0 | 0 |

However, when compared to coconut oil, coconut meat looks incredibly nutritious. Calorie for calorie, coconut meat contains eight times more vitamin E. Coconut oil is almost completely devoid of every other essential nutrient, except for the omega-6 essential fat linoleic acid. A day's worth of calories from coconut oil would barely provide the required amount. As this model demonstrates, the whole food is much more nutritious than the processed food.

Olives and olive oil are also popular foods in some camps of the raw-food community. Olives are a high-fat food, with comparatively less carbohydrate and much less protein relative to its fat content. But olives actually do have some carbohydrate and protein, while olive oil has none. Three-quarters of a cup of olives has a similar number of calories to one tablespoon of olive oil!

Olives are not a good source of most vitamins, with the exception of beta-carotene—not surprising, given that beta-carotene is a fat-soluble phytonutrient and olives are high in fat. The nutrient analysis of olive oil indicates that there is no beta-carotene in the sample of extravirgin olive oil tested.

There are small amounts of a few vitamins and minerals in this sample of olive oil. The calcium and iron content of the olives is surprising, especially the iron. There are far fewer minerals in the olive oil, as it appears that most of the minerals are not retained in the oil-pressing process.

**Table 11.2.** A comparison of the nutrients in extra-virgin olive oil and black olives

| Nutrient | Olive oil (1 Tbsp/13.5 g) | Olives (¾ c/100.8 g) |
|---|---|---|
| Calories (kcal) | 119 | 116 |
| Carbohydrate (g) | 0 | 6.3 |
| Protein (g) | 0 | 0.9 |
| Fat (g) | 13.5 | 10.8 |
| Percentage of calories from fat | 100 | 84 |
| Saturated fat (g) | 1.9 | 1.4 |
| Monounsaturated fat (g) | 9.9 | 8 |
| Polyunsaturated fat (g) | 1.4 | 0.9 |

| Vitamins | | | Adult DRI |
|---|---|---|---|
| A (RAE) | 0 | 20 | 700–900 |
| Beta-carotene (mcg) | 0 | 239 | - |
| $B_1$ (mg) | 0 | 0 | 1.1–1.2 |
| $B_2$ (mg) | 0 | 0 | 1.1–1.3 |
| $B_3$ (mg) | 0 | 0.04 | 14–16 |
| $B_5$ (mg) | 0 | 0.02 | 5 |
| $B_6$ (mg) | 0 | 0.01 | 1.3–1.7 |
| Folate/$B_9$ (mcg) | 0 | 0 | 400 |
| $B_{12}$ (mcg) | 0 | 0 | 2.4 |
| C (mg) | 0 | 0.91 | 75–90 |
| D (IU) | 0 | 0 | 600–800 |
| E (mg) | 1.94 | 1.66 | 15 |

| Minerals | Olive oil (1 Tbsp/13.5 g) | Olives (¾ c/100.8 g) | Adult DRI |
|---|---|---|---|
| Calcium (mg) | 0.1 | 89 | 1,000–1,200 |
| Copper (mcg) | 0 | 250 | 900 |
| Iron (mg) | 0.1 | 3.3 | 8–18 |
| Magnesium (mg) | 0 | 4 | 310–420 |
| Manganese (mg) | 0 | 0.02 | 1.8–2.3 |
| Potassium (mg) | 0.1 | 8.1 | 4,700 |
| Selenium (mcg) | 0 | 0.9 | 55 |
| Sodium (mg) | 0.3 | 879 | 1,200–1,500 |
| Zinc (mg) | 0 | 0.2 | 8–11 |

| Amino acids | | |
|---|---|---|
| Histidine (g) | 0 | 0.02 |
| Isoleucine (g) | 0 | 0.03 |
| Leucine (g) | 0 | 0.05 |
| Lysine (g) | 0 | 0.03 |
| Methionine (+ cysteine) (g) | 0 | 0.01 |
| Phenylalanine (+ tyrosine) (g) | 0 | 0.05 |
| Threonine (g) | 0 | 0.03 |
| Tryptophan (g) | 0 | Not reported |
| Valine (g) | 0 | 0.04 |
| **Saturated fatty acids** | | |
| Palmitic acid (g) | 1.52 | 1.19 |
| Stearic acid (g) | 0.26 | 0.24 |
| **Polyunsaturated fatty acids** | | |
| Linoleic acid (LA) omega-6 (g) | 1.32 | 0.85 |
| Alpha-linolenic acid (ALA) omega-3 (g) | 0.10 | 0.06 |
| Eicosapentaenoic acid (EPA) omega-3 (g) | 0 | 0 |
| Docosahexaenoic acid (DHA) omega-3 (g) | 0 | 0 |
| **Monounsaturated fatty acids** | | |
| Oleic acid, omega-9 (g) | 9.62 | 7.95 |

The difference between a whole food and its processed derivative becomes even more striking when looking at flaxseeds and flax oil. The calorie equivalent of 1 tablespoon of flax oil is 2 tablespoons of flaxseeds. As shown in table 11.3, the vitamin content of flaxseeds (with the exception of vitamins $B_{12}$ and D) is worthy of consideration, particularly vitamin $B_1$ (thiamin). It appears that the vitamin content of flaxseeds is not retained in flax oil. The mineral content of flaxseeds is considerable, while the mineral content of flax oil is negligible. As with all other oils, there is no protein in flax oil.

The oil doesn't contain notable amounts of any essential nutrients, with the exception of the omega-3 essential fat alpha-linolenic acid (ALA). For the same number of calories, the flax oil has more ALA than flaxseeds because flaxseeds also have protein and carbohydrate. The omega-6 to omega-3 ratio of about 1:4 is excellent for both flaxseeds and flax oil.

**Table 11.3.** A comparison of the nutrients in flax oil and flaxseeds

| Nutrient | Flax oil (1 Tbsp/13.6 g) | Flaxseeds, golden (2 Tbsp/20.6 g) |
|---|---|---|
| Calories (kcal) | 120 | 120 |
| Carbohydrate (g) | 0 | 6.5 g |
| Protein (g) | 0 | 4.1 g |
| Fat (g) | 13.6 g | 9.5 g |
| Percentage of calories from fat | 100 | 71 |
| Saturated fat (g) | 1.3 g | 0.8 g |
| Monounsaturated fat (g) | 2.8 g | 1.7 g |
| Polyunsaturated fat (g) | 9.0 g | 6.34 g |

| Vitamins | | | Adult DRI |
|---|---|---|---|
| A (RAE) | 0 | 0 | 700–900 |
| Beta-carotene (mcg) | 0 | 0 | - |
| $B_1$ (mg) | 0 | 0.4 | 1.1–1.2 |
| $B_2$ (mg) | 0 | 0.1 | 1.1–1.3 |
| $B_3$ (mg) | 0 | 0.7 | 14–16 |
| $B_5$ (mg) | 0 | 0.2 | 5 |
| $B_6$ (mg) | 0 | 0.1 | 1.3–1.7 |
| Folate/$B_9$ (mcg) | 0 | 19.6 | 400 |
| $B_{12}$ (mcg) | 0 | 0 | 2.4 |
| C (mg) | 0 | 0.1 | 75–90 |
| D (IU) | 0 | 0 | 600–800 |
| E (mg) | 2.4 | 0.1 | 15 |

| Minerals | Flax oil (1 Tbsp/13.6 g) | Flaxseeds, golden (2 Tbsp/20.6 g) | Adult DRI |
|---|---|---|---|
| Calcium (mg) | 0 | 57 | 1,000–1,200 |
| Copper (mcg) | 0 | 270 | 900 |
| Iron (mg) | 0 | 1.3 | 8–18 |
| Magnesium (mg) | 0 | 89 | 310–420 |
| Manganese (mg) | 0 | 0.6 | 1.8–2.3 |
| Potassium (mg) | 0 | 183 | 4,700 |
| Selenium (mcg) | 0 | 5.7 | 55 |
| Sodium (mg) | 0 | 6.7 | 1,200–1,500 |
| Zinc (mg) | 0 | 1 | 8–11 |

| Amino acids | | |
|---|---|---|
| Histidine (g) | 0 | 0.10 |
| Isoleucine (g) | 0 | 0.19 |
| Leucine (g) | 0 | 0.26 |
| Lysine (g) | 0 | 0.18 |
| Methionine (+ cysteine) (g) | 0 | 0.15 |
| Phenylalanine (+ tyrosine) (g) | 0 | 0.30 |
| Threonine (g) | 0 | 0.16 |
| Tryptophan (g) | 0 | 0.06 |
| Valine (g) | 0 | 0.22 |
| **Saturated fatty acids** | | |
| Palmitic acid (g) | 0.72 | 0.49 |
| Stearic acid (g) | 0.56 | 0.30 |
| **Polyunsaturated fatty acids** | | |
| Linoleic acid (LA) omega-6 (g) | 1.73 | 1.33 |
| Alpha-linolenic acid (ALA) omega-3 (g) | 7.25 | 5.13 |
| Eicosapentaenoic acid (EPA) omega-3 (g) | 0 | 0 |
| Docosahexaenoic acid (DHA) omega-3 (g) | 0 | 0 |
| **Monounsaturated fatty acids** | | |
| Oleic acid omega-9 (g) | 2.75 | 1.69 |

Chia seeds also have an impressive nutritional profile, especially when compared to chia seed oil. Two tablespoons of chia seeds contain almost four grams of protein, a notable amount. There is no protein in chia seed oil. Although the only vitamin reported in the seeds is $B_3$ (niacin), no vitamins are reported in chia oil. The calcium content of chia seeds is significant, almost 160 milligrams for about 2 tablespoons. No minerals are reported for chia seed oil.

The omega-6 to omega-3 ratio of chia seeds shown by this data is excellent—1:3. Because oil is a concentrated source of fats, the omega-6 to omega-3 content and ratio of chia seed oil is also excellent—1:3.3. But overall, the whole seeds bring so much more to the table.

**Table 11.4.** A comparison of the nutrients in chia seed oil and chia seeds

| Nutrient | Chia seed oil (1 Tbsp/14 g) | Chia seeds (2 Tbsp/20 g) |
|---|---|---|
| Calories (kcal) | 130 | 120 |
| Carbohydrate (g) | 0 | 10.7 |
| Protein (g) | 0 | 3.8 |
| Fat (g) | 14 | 7.5 |
| Percentage of calories from fat | 100 | 56 |
| Saturated fat (g) | 1.5 | 0.8 |
| Monounsaturated fat (g) | 1 | 0.5 |
| Polyunsaturated fat (g) | 11.5 | 5.7 |

| Vitamins | | | Adult DRI |
|---|---|---|---|
| $B_3$ (mg) | 0 | 2.6 | 14–16 |
| **Minerals** | | | |
| Calcium (mg) | 0 | 160 | 1,000–1,200 |
| Copper (mcg) | 0 | 50 | 900 |
| Manganese (mg) | 0 | 0.5 | 1.8–2.3 |
| Potassium (mg) | 0 | 39.2 | 4,700 |
| Sodium (mg) | 0 | 4.6 | 1,200–1,500 |
| Zinc (mg) | 0 | 0.86 | 8–11 |

| Amino acids | | |
|---|---|---|
| Histidine (g) | 0 | 0.11 |
| Isoleucine (g) | 0 | 0.15 |
| Leucine (g) | 0 | 0.27 |
| Lysine (g) | 0 | 0.20 |
| Methionine (+ cysteine) (g) | 0 | 0.10 |
| Phenylalanine (+ tyrosine) (g) | 0 | 0.33 |

| Amino acids | Chia seed oil (1 Tbsp/14 g) | Chia seeds (2 Tbsp/20 g) |
|---|---|---|
| Threonine (g) | 0 | 0.14 |
| Tryptophan (g) | 0 | 0.16 |
| Valine (g) | 0 | 0.23 |
| **Saturated fatty acids** | | |
| Palmitic acid 16:1 | Not available | 0.50 g |
| Stearic acid 18:0 | Not available | 0.22 g |
| **Polyunsaturated fatty acids** | | |
| Linoleic acid (LA) omega-6 (g) | 2.690 | 1.42 |
| Alpha-linolenic acid (ALA) omega-3 (g) | 8.77 | 4.30 |
| Eicosapentaenoic acid (EPA) omega-3 (g) | 0 | 0 |
| Docosahexaenoic acid (DHA) omega-3 (g) | 0 | 0 |
| **Monounsaturated fatty acids** | | |
| Oleic acid, omega-9 (g) | 1 | 0.49 |

## Popular Raw Food Sweeteners

Another trend in some camps of the raw-food community is the use of sweeteners, such as agave syrup (nectar), yacon syrup, Jerusalem artichoke sugar, coconut sugar, and others. These concentrated sweeteners are all derived from whole plant foods. Just as with oil, I believe that these sweeteners may have their place, such as in celebratory situations or for people transitioning from a standard Western diet. However, having whole foods as the major focus of the diet will provide the greatest nutrient content per calorie.

Table 11.5 shows that agave syrup is virtually 100-percent carbohydrate, similar to how the various oils that we discussed are 100-percent fat. The measured calorie content of 18 grams of dried edible portion of agave plant is equivalent to about 64 calories of agave syrup. The vitamin content of agave syrup is higher than dried agave for some vitamins and lower for others. The overall vitamin content of both foods is unremarkable. The mineral content of dried agave is substantial, especially for calcium and zinc, but that of agave syrup is negligible. Again, the whole food is a pretty solid source of many nutrients and fiber, while the extracted, processed food provides a concentrated source of largely empty calories.

People ask me what I use to sweeten recipes, for example, in tomato sauce and salad dressing, and the answer is some type of whole fruit, usually dates. Table 11.6 on page 158 gives the nutrient content of several samples of sweet fruits with a similar calorie level as the dried agave and agave syrup in table 11.5.

Compared to agave syrup, strawberries clearly are winners. The daily value for vitamin C can be achieved with this amount of strawberries alone. Raspberries are clearly superior to agave syrup in mineral content, and figs are an impressive source of calcium. Like raspberries, medjool dates are more mineral-rich than agave syrup.

Without a doubt, the fruits shown here are much richer sources of nutrients than agave syrup. Raw-food enthusiasts who rely on sweeteners such as agave syrup may not get as many nutrients overall as they would by consuming whole fruits.

## Why Eating More Whole Foods Leads to Success

I've heard people say that a vegan diet didn't work for them, but when I looked closely at what they actually ate, there were contributing factors that weren't necessarily related to veganism. Not all vegan diets are identical, and neither are all omnivorous diets. Some of the factors that will derail any dietary approach include the following:

- not focusing on whole foods as the primary source of calories and overconsuming empty calories, such as oil and isolated sweeteners
- not eating enough calories

**Table 11.5.** A comparison of the nutrients in agave syrup and dried agave

| Nutrient | Agave syrup (1 Tbsp/21g) | Agave, dried (18 g) |
|---|---|---|
| Calories (kcal) | 64 | 61 |
| Carbohydrate (g) | 15.8 | 14.8 |
| Protein (g) | 0.02 | 0.31 |
| Fat (g) | 0.1 | 0.1 |
| Dietary fiber (g) | 0 | 2.8 |

| **Vitamins** | | | Adult DRI |
|---|---|---|---|
| A (RAE) | 2 | 0.2 | 700–900 |
| Beta-carotene (mcg) | 0 | 2 | - |
| B$_1$ (mg) | 0.03 | 0.01 | 1.1–1.2 |
| B$_2$ (mg) | 0.03 | 0.1 | 1.1–1.3 |
| B$_3$ (mg) | 0.14 | 0.2 | 14–16 |
| B$_5$ (mg) | Not available | 0.1 | 5 |
| B$_6$ (mg) | 0.05 | 0.1 | 1.3–1.7 |
| Folate/B$_9$ (mcg) | Not available | 1.3 | 400 |
| B$_{12}$ (mcg) | 0 | 0 | 2.4 |
| C (mg) | 3.5 | 0.1 | 75–90 |
| D (IU) | 0 | 0 | 600–800 |
| E (mg) | 0.2 | 0.1 | 15 |

| Minerals | Agave syrup (1 Tbsp/21g) | Agave, dried (18 g) | Adult DRI |
|---|---|---|---|
| Calcium (mg) | 0 | 139 | 1,000–1,200 |
| Iron (mg) | 0.02 | 0.7 | 8–18 |
| Magnesium (mg) | 0 | 37.3 | 310–420 |
| Potassium (mg) | 1 | 138 | 4,700 |
| Sodium (mg) | 1 | 3 | 1,200–1,500 |
| Zinc (mg) | 0 | 2.2 | 8–11 |

It's not enough just to eat raw food ingredients in any quantity with a lack of regard for their nutritional content. Lack of proper nutrition education may have led to many nutritional myths in the raw-food community. These include the notions that a raw dessert is a nutritionally superior breakfast food, any one particular superfood needs to be consumed every day, leafy greens are expendable, all fruits are bad, all high-fat foods are bad, the consumption of raw oils is essential, one can get enough calories from vegetables and sprouts alone, and that eating a large salad is impossible.

For instance, some people won't eat fruit because of the inaccurate perception that it's high glycemic, yet be perfectly fine with eating raw desserts containing concentrated sweeteners. To get another sense of how the nutri-

**Table 11.6.** A comparison of the nutrients in a variety of fruits

| Nutrient | Strawberries (1⅛ c, sliced/187 g) | Raspberries (1 c/123 g) | Figs (2, fresh/ 102 g) | Medjool dates (1, pitted/ 24 g) |
|---|---|---|---|---|
| Calories (kcal) | 60 | 64 | 74 | 66 |
| Carbohydrate (g) | 14.3 | 14.7 | 18.7 | 18 |
| Protein (g) | 1.3 | 1.5 | 0.7 | 0.4 |
| Fat (g) | 0.6 | 0.8 | 0.30 | 0.1 |
| Dietary fiber (g) | 3.7 | 8 | 2.7 | 1.6 |

| Vitamins | | | | | Adult DRI |
|---|---|---|---|---|---|
| Vitamin A (RAE) | 1.1 | 2 | 6.7 | 1.8 | 700–900 |
| Beta-carotene (mcg) | 13.1 | 14.8 | 13.3 | 21.4 | - |
| B₁ (mg) | 0.04 | 0.04 | 0.06 | 0.01 | 1.1–1.2 |
| B₂ (mg) | 0.04 | 0.05 | 0.05 | 0.01 | 1.1–1.3 |

| Vitamins | Strawberries (1⅛ c, sliced/187 g) | Raspberries (1 c/123 g) | Figs (2, fresh/ 102 g) | Medjool dates (1, pitted/ 24 g) | Adult DRI |
|---|---|---|---|---|---|
| $B_3$ (mg) | 0.72 | 0.74 | 0.40 | 0.39 | 14–16 |
| $B_5$ (mg) | 0.23 | 0.40 | Not available | 0.19 | 5 |
| $B_6$ (mg) | 0.09 | 0.07 | 0.11 | 0.06 | 1.3–1.7 |
| Folate/$B_9$ (mcg) | 44.8 | 25.8 | 6 | 3.6 | 400 |
| $B_{12}$ (mcg) | 0 | 0 | 0 | 0 | 2.4 |
| C (mg) | 110 | 32 | 2.4 | 0 | 75–90 |
| D (IU) | 0 | 0 | 0 | 0 | 600–800 |
| E (mg) | 0.5 | 1.1 | 0.1 | Not available | 15 |
| **Minerals** | | | | | |
| Calcium (mg) | 30 | 31 | 40 | 15 | 1,000– 1,200 |
| Iron (mg) | 0.8 | 0.9 | 0.4 | 0.2 | 8–18 |
| Magnesium (mg) | 24 | 27 | 17 | 13 | 310–420 |
| Potassium (mg) | 286 | 186 | 232 | 167 | 4,700 |
| Sodium (mg) | 1.9 | 1.2 | 1 | 0.2 | 1,200–1,500 |
| Zinc (mg) | 0.3 | 0.5 | 0.2 | 0.11 | 8–11 |

ents in whole foods stack up against those in raw ingredients that have been derived from whole foods, let's compare two popular raw foods shown on page 161: a green fruit smoothie and a piece of raw chocolate pie.

Because of its fruit content, the smoothie is high in carbohydrate, and the amount of nuts and seeds in the pie slice contributes to the high percentage of calories from fat. Even though both recipes contain a similar number of calories, the green smoothie provides impressive amounts of B vitamins—close to half the adult daily values for many of them with the exception of vitamin $B_{12}$. The daily value of vitamin C has been exceeded by a long shot and the beta-carotene content is also high.

The piece of pie has a decent B-vitamin content (again with the exception of vitamin $B_{12}$) and the vitamin E content is also especially good. However, the levels of B vitamins in the green smoothie are superior to those of the pie. The vitamin C content of the green smoothie is also much better than that of the pie, as is the beta-carotene content. The pie does beat the green smoothie with one vitamin—vitamin E—given that vitamin E is fat-soluble and there's much more fat in the pie than in the smoothie. Beta-carotene is also fat-soluble, but it's mostly found in fruits and vegetables, which would account for its content in the green smoothie and lack thereof in the slice of pie.

The mineral content of this smoothie is impressive, especially the calcium, iron, and potassium content. The mineral profile of the pie slice is strong in many instances, but the green smoothie is superior in calcium, potassium, and manganese. The pie has more iron and zinc, which mostly come from the cashews and almonds. These two nuts are really the most nutrient-dense ingredients in this piece of pie.

With its high vitamin and mineral content, the smoothie is clearly more nutrient dense than the piece of pie. Desserts can still have a place in a nutritious diet. If someone is struggling to eat a healthy diet and it's easier for them to maintain (without significant backsliding or giving up altogether) if they're able to eat a piece of raw pie once in a while, then having occasional treats may be helpful for that person at that point in time. As long as high-fat, high-calorie, lower-nutrient foods don't regularly take the place of more nutrient-dense foods, I'm very much in favor of people finding a sustainable approach that gives them the health results they're seeking. Another important consideration is how a person feels after they eat. In this case, some people may feel much more energetic after consuming the green smoothie than after eating the pie. Personal experience and results along with nutrient information can help someone make food choices that are the best for them.

**Table 11.7.** A comparison of a green smoothie and slice of raw chocolate pie

| Nutrients | Green smoothie | Raw chocolate pie, 1 slice |
|---|---|---|
| Calories (kcal) | 740 | 741 |
| Carbohydrate as a percentage of calories | 87 | 25 |
| Protein as a percentage of calories | 8 | 10 |
| Fat as a percentage of calories | 5 | 65 |
| Saturated fat (g) | 0.7 | 12.6 |

| Vitamins | | | Adult DRI |
|---|---|---|---|
| A (RAE) | 1,073 | 0.1 | 700–900 |
| Beta-carotene (mcg) | 12,710 | 1.6 | - |
| $B_1$ (mg) | 0.6 | 0.3 | 1.1–1.2 |
| $B_2$ (mg) | 0.7 | 0.5 | 1.1–1.3 |
| $B_3$ (mg) | 6.7 | 2.5 | 14–16 |

| Vitamins | Green smoothie | Raw chocolate pie, 1 slice | Adult DRI |
|---|---|---|---|
| B₅ (mg) | 2.5 | 0.8 | 5 |
| B₆ (mg) | 2.1 | 0.3 | 1.3–1.7 |
| Folate/B₉ (mcg) | 259 | 40.6 | 400 |
| B₁₂ (mcg) | 0 | 0 | 2.4 |
| C (mg) | 504 | 0.3 | 75–90 |
| D (IU) | 0 | 0 | 600–800 |
| E (mg) | 3.3 | 12.5 | 15 |
| **Minerals** | | | |
| Calcium (mg) | 344 | 156 | 1,000–1,200 |
| Copper (mcg) | 1,070 | 1,774 | 900 |
| Iron (mg) | 5.5 | 5.8 | 8–18 |
| Magnesium (mg) | 218 | 298 | 310–420 |
| Manganese (mg) | 4.2 | 2.1 | 1.8–2.3 |
| Potassium (mg) | 2915 | 848 | 4,700 |
| Selenium (mcg) | 7.2 | 11.9 | 55 |
| Sodium (mg) | 67 | 8 | 1,200–1,500 |
| Zinc (mg) | 2.2 | 4.6 | 8–11 |

Here's a comparison of the calories in the green smoothie versus the piece of raw pie:

### Green Smoothie (740 calories)

2 cups (134 g) chopped kale

1½ medium (182 g) oranges

2 cups (296 g) fresh blueberries

3 medium (236 g) bananas

2 cups (332 g) fresh strawberries, halved

### Raw Chocolate Pie, 1 slice (741 calories)

Crust

⅓ cup (48 g) almonds

2 tablespoons (18 g) chopped deglet noor dates

Filling

⅓ cup (47 g) cashews

1 tablespoon (21 g) agave syrup

1 tablespoon (5.4 g) cacao powder

1 teaspoon (4.5 g) cacao butter

1 teaspoon (4.7 g) coconut oil

½ teaspoon (2.1 g) vanilla extract

As you can see, this pie slice, just as with similar desserts, is high in calories. Many people may not realize this. Since the pie slice is so high in calories, I created a green smoothie recipe with a similar number of calories for a per-calorie comparison of the two.

It's revealing to compare this slice of pie to the large vegetable garden salad shown on the facing page and in table 11.8. This salad is a modified version of the 611-calorie salad on page 123. The pie and salad have similar calorie contents; however, the pie slice is very calorie dense and not as nutrient dense as the salad. The salad, on the other hand, is not very calorie dense and contains impressive amounts of important nutrients, for only 738 calories. It has more than the adult daily value for vitamins $B_1$, $B_2$, $B_6$, C, and E and folate. Beta-carotene content is excellent and vitamins $B_3$ and $B_5$ are close to their respective daily values. Calorie for calorie, this salad is the most vitamin dense, followed by the green smoothie, then the slice of pie. The salad also contains notable amounts of minerals, with the adult daily values exceeded for potassium, copper, and manganese. The calcium, iron, magnesium, and zinc content is excellent. Celery, Swiss chard, and bok choy are notable whole-food sources of sodium.

**Table 11.8.** Nutrient content of salad and dressing compared to slice of raw chocolate pie

| Nutrients | Salad and dressing | Raw chocolate pie, 1 slice |
|---|---|---|
| Calories (kcal) | 738 | 741 |
| Carbohydrate as a percentage of calories | 48 | 25 |
| Protein as a percentage of calories | 17 | 10 |
| Fat as a percentage of calories | 35 | 65 |
| Saturated fat (g) | 3.3 | 12.6 |

| Vitamins | | | Adult DRI |
|---|---|---|---|
| A (RAE) | 4,721 | 0.1 | 700–900 |
| Beta-carotene (mcg) | 53,625 | 1.6 | - |
| $B_1$ (mg) | 1.4 | 0.3 | 1.1–1.2 |
| $B_2$ (mg) | 1.7 | 0.5 | 1.1–1.3 |
| $B_3$ (mg) | 11.2 | 2.5 | 14–16 |
| $B_5$ (mg) | 3.4 | 0.8 | 5 |
| $B_6$ (mg) | 2.7 | 0.3 | 1.3–1.7 |
| Folate/$B_9$ (mcg) | 1,189 | 40.6 | 400 |

| Vitamins | Salad and dressing | Raw chocolate pie, 1 slice | Adult DRI |
|---|---|---|---|
| B₁₂ (mcg) | 0 | 0 | 2.4 |
| C (mg) | 697 | 0.3 | 75–90 |
| D (IU) | 0 | 0 | 600–800 |
| E (mg) | 15.9 | 12.5 | 15 |
| **Minerals** | | | |
| Calcium (mg) | 883 | 156 | 1,000–1,200 |
| Copper (mcg) | 1,880 | 1,774 | 900 |
| Iron (mg) | 17 | 5.8 | 8–18 |
| Magnesium (mg) | 373 | 298 | 310–420 |
| Manganese (mg) | 3.8 | 2.1 | 1.8–2.3 |
| Potassium (mg) | 4,704 | 848 | 4,700 |
| Selenium (mcg) | 6.1 | 11.9 | 55 |
| Sodium (mg) | 258 | 8 | 1,200–1,500 |
| Zinc (mg) | 6.8 | 4.6 | 8–11 |

I've observed that getting selenium can be challenging on raw food diets and other dietary approaches, and one Brazil nut can account for more than the daily value. Consuming adequate amounts of vitamins $B_{12}$ and D can be a challenge for anyone, regardless of diet.

### Salad and Dressing (738 calories)
Salad
1 head (626 g) romaine lettuce, chopped
4 cups (99 g) chopped dandelion greens
1 cup (180 g) chopped tomatoes
1 cup (104 g) chopped cucumber
1 cup (110 g) grated carrots
¼ cup (37.5 g) sliced Jerusalem artichokes

Salad Dressing
2 cups (298 g) chopped red bell pepper
2 cups (248 g) chopped zucchini
½ cup (122 g) fresh-squeezed lemon juice
2 tablespoons (18 g) almonds
2 tablespoons (20 g) chia seeds
2 tablespoons (18 g) unhulled sesame seeds

The bottom line is that when components of food are removed from their whole-food matrix, the food is altered in many ways, including its nutrient content. The greatest relevance this has for someone on a raw food diet is the use of oil and sweeteners. Making nutrient comparisons like the ones in this chapter is a great way to help someone make the very best choices.

## CHAPTER 12
# Principles of Food Combining

B EFORE I STARTED ON MY PATH TO HEALTH, I never really considered the effect that food had on my body, nor was I aware of the differences that food made to my health. In fact, I never even thought much about food beyond taste and convention. It wasn't until my health had declined to a point I could no longer accept that I started looking for unconventional solutions. After I incorporated more raw foods into my diet, I finally realized how good I could actually feel and how much energy I could experience.

I noticed that when I changed my diet, my body became more attuned to what I was eating. I noticed that when I ate lighter raw foods, my body felt more energetic, whereas when I ate heavier or more cooked or processed foods, I didn't have as much energy. Not everyone has the same reaction, but overall, I'd say that most people with whom I've spoken about this do notice a difference.

There are basic principles of health that apply to any eating pattern. Within that framework, however, there's quite a bit of room for variation. Each individual needs to engage in some personal experimentation to observe which pieces of the overall health puzzle are more or less relevant for them.

## The Basic Principles of Food Combining

One of the things I've noticed in my personal health journey is that eating fruits at a different time than other foods helps my digestion, while if I eat fruits on top of cooked foods or more dense raw foods, I feel less energetic. This experience is consistent with the principles of food combining, an approach to eating that suggests which foods should or shouldn't be eaten at the same meal to enhance the digestive process. Most of the information available on food combining is from anecdotal experience, and there's little peer-reviewed research in this area. However, it's difficult to discount what works for someone, myself included.

The idea of grouping foods according to their perceived macronutrient content to determine when to eat them has been outlined in raw-food books written by popular authors, such as Herbert Shelton and Ann Wigmore. Generally, the foods are grouped as follows, but there's not absolute agreement as to which foods belong in each group.

Fruits
- acid fruits (grapefruit, lemons, limes, oranges, pineapples, strawberries, tomatoes)

- sub-acid fruits (apples, berries, cherries, grapes, peaches, pears, plums, other stone fruits)
- sweet fruits (bananas, dates, dried fruits, figs, papayas, persimmons)
- melons (cantaloupes, honeydew, watermelons)

Proteins
- legumes and lentils (beans, lentils, peanuts, peas, soy)
- nuts and seeds (almonds, Brazil nuts, cashews, flaxseeds, pumpkin seeds, sesame seeds, sunflower seeds, walnuts)
- animal products, for people who consume them (cheese, eggs, fish, poultry, meat, milk)

Starches and starchy vegetables
- grains (bread, corn, millet, oats, pasta, rice, rye, wheat)
- pseudograins (amaranth, buckwheat, quinoa)
- roots and tubers (carrots, parsnips, sweet potatoes, white potatoes, yams)
- starchy vegetables (winter squash, pumpkins)

Low-starch vegetables
- leafy greens (bok choy, chard, collard greens, kale, lettuce, dandelion greens, napa cabbage)
- other vegetables (beets, broccoli, celery, cucumbers, eggplant, jicama, radishes, red peppers, sprouts, summer squash, zucchini)

Fats and oils
- high-fat foods (avocados, butter, coconut, cream)
- vegetable, nut, and seed oils (canola, coconut, corn, olive, sesame, and sunflower oils and margarine)

According to some food-combining philosophies, each category of food requires a different type of enzyme for digestion. They assert that protein foods require a protein-digesting enzyme, fatty foods require a fat-digesting enzyme, and starches require a starch-digesting enzyme. According to proponents of these philosophies, the digestive tract secretes these enzymes specifically for the food that is present at the time. When there are two conflicting types of foods present, the digestive tract will release enzymes for these specific foods, and these conflicting enzymes effectively cancel each other out in the digestive system and render them ineffective, leading to gas, bloating, and indigestion.

Some promoters of food combining recognize three phases of food metabolism:

- digestion: noon to 8 p.m.
- assimilation: 8 p.m. to 4 a.m.
- elimination: 4 a.m. to noon

Others take this concept a step further and state that no food should be consumed before noon to maximize detoxification and elimination, but this approach may not be suitable for everyone. All generally agree that someone should eat when hungry, chew food well, and not overeat.

## Principles of Combining Fruits

Of all the categories, the most guidelines or rules have been written about how and when to consume fruits. Given the perception that fruits are digested relatively quickly and easily, fruits are ideally the only foods to be eaten before noon to allow the body to focus on elimination.

The following principles govern when to eat fruits and how to eat them with other foods:

- Fruits are best eaten alone and on an empty stomach and should be given 30 to 60 minutes to digest before consuming the next course.
- Fruits are thought to move more quickly through the digestive tract than proteins, fats, starches, and vegetables.
- Eating fruits with proteins, fats, or starches slows down the digestive process.
- Fruits contain simple carbohydrates that digest more quickly than foods that contain more complex carbohydrates, such as fructose, glucose, and sucrose.

The following principles guide how to eat specific fruits:

- Melons are best eaten separately from other fruits.
- Fruits are best not eaten for dessert or right after a meal consisting of other foods.
- Sub-acid fruits, such as apples and pears, may be eaten with sweet fruits, such as dates and bananas, or acid fruits, such as citrus.
- Sweet fruits and acid fruits are best not eaten together.
- Low-sugar fruits, such as tomatoes, lemons, and limes, can be eaten with greens and other salad vegetables, but not starchy vegetables, such as carrots.
- Cooked foods are not to be eaten with fruits and fruits are not to be cooked.

### Principles of Combining Leafy Green Vegetables
- Leafy greens can be eaten with either starches or proteins, but not both.
- Cooked or dehydrated foods are best eaten with a vegetable salad.

### Principles of Combining Protein, Starch, and Fat
- Starchy vegetables are not to be mixed with nuts or seeds.
- Fats combine well with proteins, starches, or nonstarchy vegetables.

## What Researchers Say about Food Combining

Although these food-combining concepts have been followed rigorously by their proponents for almost a century, rarely has anyone challenged the science behind them. We'll review the most popular concepts and see if they hold up to scientific scrutiny.

### Three Phases of Food Metabolism

The processes of digestion, assimilation, elimination, and detoxification all occur at the same time and whenever they're needed. So far there's no information substantiating the claim that each of these processes is dominant at specified times. On the other hand, some people do notice a difference when consuming foods at certain times of the day, such as eating lighter foods before noon. Although eating exclusively fruits before noon or not consuming any food before noon may be helpful for some, this is not an approach that necessarily works for everyone.

### Rates of Digestion

Fruits are thought to move more quickly through the digestive tract than other foods because of their simple carbohydrate content. However, as we saw in table 1.1 (pages 6–7), most fruits do contain some protein and fat, although they're mainly composed of the simple sugars fructose and glucose. Because these simple sugars don't need to be broken down further by enzymes in order to be absorbed, some food-combining advocates refer to fruit as being "predigested." Could this predigested state cause fruit to move more quickly through the digestive tract? No specific studies measure the digestive processing of fruit versus other foods, so the information on this is currently incomplete.

However, the idea that fruit is more quickly digested than other foods is challenged by the data that we have on blood sugar. Some researchers suggest that an easily digested food high in carbohydrates will raise blood sugar more quickly than foods that are lower on the glycemic index. For example, white bread is higher on the glycemic index than most types of fruit. Does this mean that white bread is more quickly digested in the stomach than a piece of fruit? Not necessarily. Also, fructose does not raise blood sugar as much as glucose, regardless of how quickly it is absorbed. So, perhaps blood sugar measurements or the glycemic index may not be the best indicators of how quickly fruits are digested and absorbed relative to other high-carbohydrate foods. Getting a direct measurement of how quickly individual foods are digested would be the best way to find out. In the end, personal experience can be helpful in determining what works best. Many people have reported that when they eat fruit with heavier foods (such as starches or proteins) or after a meal as a dessert, they find that their digestion is not as favorable as when they eat fruit alone. Fruit is often not a problem when mixed with low-starch vegetables, such in a green smoothie.

Absorption rates of carbohydrate, protein, and fat have been reported in some physiology textbooks, but there have been studies that have shown these rates to vary depending on a number of factors, including the content of fiber and other components in foods. Most foods contain a combination of macronutrients and other substances that may affect digestion, with the exceptions of oil (which is 100 percent fat) and some sweeteners (which are 100 percent carbohydrate).

Aspects of digestive physiology that are very well understood are the processes used by the body to directly digest carbohydrate, protein, and fat. Carbohydrate digestion involves the breakdown of more complex carbohydrates into simple carbohydrates. For instance, the complex carbohydrates found in vegetables and grains must be broken down by the enzyme amylase in order to be absorbed. The simple carbohydrates fructose and glucose, found largely in fruits, don't need to be broken down to be absorbed. We still don't know how this affects the exact rate at which these foods are digested, but we do know for sure that most vegetables and grains require more enzymes to digest than most fruits, depending on the types and amounts of carbohydrates found in individual foods.

Protein digestion requires pepsin, a protein-digesting enzyme found in the stomach, and proteases, a group of protein-digesting enzymes made by the pancreas and released into the small intestine. Fat digestion requires lipase, a fat-digesting enzyme made by the pancreas and released into the small intestine. Bile, which is also released into the small intestine in the presence of fat, emulsifies the fat, allowing lipase to digest it more easily.

Looking at this information, one might draw the conclusion that fat requires the most digestive resources, followed by protein and carbohydrates. How this translates to actual rates of digestion is yet to be fully understood.

**Enzyme Cancellation**

The enzyme cancellation concept attempts to justify the grouping and consumption of foods based on the belief that the digestive system only secretes one type of enzyme at a time. It's assumed, then, that when certain foods are eaten together, the body can't digest them because the enzymes needed to process them somehow cancel each other out. However, when food passes from the stomach into the small intestine, the pancreas actually releases all three types of digestive enzymes—amylase, protease, and lipase—at the same time. If it were the case that digestive enzymes competed with each other or cancelled each other out, no foods would ever get digested. Again, table 1.1 (pags 6–7) underscores this point, showing how whole natural plant foods contain a combination of all three macronutrients, carbohydrate, protein, and fat. Even tomatoes have a surprisingly high percentage of their calories (17 percent) from protein, for a fruit.

Numerous foods in a raw diet provide great examples of the range of macronutrients whole foods can contain. Legumes are mostly carbohydrate but have a significant percentage of calories from protein. Almonds and sesame seeds have a much greater percentage of their calories from fat than protein, as do most nuts and seeds. Grains, pseudograins, and starchy vegetables, such as yams and carrots, are largely complex carbohydrates. However, these foods also contain protein and fat, so all three types of digestive enzymes are necessary to fully digest them. The same is true even with low-starch vegetables, such as leafy greens, peppers, broccoli, and cucumbers, and high-fat whole foods, such as avocados and coconuts.

Considering that the technology for determining the nutrient content of food was in its infancy when health enthusiasts originally wrote about food combining in the early 1900s and enzymes were less well understood at that time, we have to assume that most of these theories were developed from personal experience. This can be confusing for people who take these groupings literally. I would encourage teachers of food combining to make this important distinction and see these principles as suggestions to help those with digestive challenges—not hard and fast rules that apply to all people in all circumstances.

**Digestive pH**

The concept of digestive pH maintains that different types of foods require different types of digestive environments. Assertions are that proteins require an acidic environment to be digested, while carbohydrates and fats require an alkaline environment. The pH scale measures how acid or alkaline a substance is; on a scale from 0 to 14, a neutral environment is 7, with substances becoming more acid as they approach 0 and more alkaline as they approach 14.

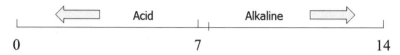

**Figure 12.1.** The pH scale

Digestion begins in the mouth with the carbohydrate-digesting enzyme amylase and fat-digesting enzyme lingual lipase. The pH of saliva generally ranges from 6 to 7. This suggests that carbohydrates and fats can be digested in a slightly acid to a neutral environment. The stomach has a pH range of 1 to 3.5, which falls well within the acid range. This environment is produced primarily by hydrochloric acid, which is needed to convert pepsinogen into the enzyme pepsin, which digests protein.

After being processed in the stomach, food moves into the small intestine. The pH of the first part of the small intestine is reported as 6, which is still in the acid range, but much less acidic than the stomach. The pancreas secretes the three types of digestive enzymes into the small intestine, along with an alkaline substance called bicarbonate to help neutralize the acid from the stomach and continue the digestive process. All three of these enzymes digest their respective macronutrients in the small intestine, so carbohydrate, protein, and fat are digested in a slightly acid environment. As food moves further into the small intestine, the pH changes to a range of 7 to 8. The enzymes that digest carbohydrate, protein, and fat are still working on their respective macronutrients, so at this point carbohydrate, protein, and fat are also digested in a neutral to slightly alkaline environment.

**Table 12.1.** Areas of the digestive tract and their respective pH ranges

| Body fluid | pH |
|---|---|
| Saliva | 6.0–7.0 |
| Gastric secretion (stomach) | 1.0–3.5 |
| Pancreatic secretion | 8.0–8.3 |

In summary, as long as the necessary digestive factors are present, all three macronutrients are digested in a range of acid/alkaline environments. Both carbohydrate and fat can be digested within a pH of 6 to 8, and protein can be digested within a range of 1 to 8.

## Food Combining and Timing: What Works

When it comes to food combining, do what works best for you. Many of our students and other people we have worked with over the years have found that certain aspects of food combining work for them, the most popular being the eating of fruit separate from heavier foods. Another popular observation is that eating a salad prior to dehydrated or cooked foods has been helpful for some people.

Aspects of food combining or the entire food-combining system may have value for some people, though not specifically for the reasons stated by some food-combining advocates. This being said, there is still much we have to learn about rates of digestion. Perhaps there are other reasons why some people get positive results from food combining; meals constructed along food-combining principles tend to be simpler, and for this reason these meals may be more easily digested.

Many people with whom we have worked have noted that they find the principles of food combining to be somewhat cumbersome. They feel pressure to follow them perfectly, especially if they're new to healthy eating and are trying to make changes to improve on past practices. This adherence may be counterproductive. We know people who have given up healthy eating completely, because they thought there were too many rules and it became too difficult to follow them. When someone is trying in earnest to make meaningful changes to their diet, the last thing they need is more hurdles in their way, especially if those hurdles aren't the most important considerations. If people abandon healthy eating because it's too difficult, they don't get any of the benefits, and that's unfortunate. It's important to note that healthful eating is a journey of self-discovery that may not conform to someone else's rules. We've noted that the people who've been the most successful in achieving their health goals were open minded and flexible in their approach, evaluated if the approach was working for them, were open to making changes, and enjoyed the process.

## CHAPTER 13

# Raw for Life: Helpful Raw-Food Success Strategies

WHETHER YOU'RE JUST STARTING A RAW FOOD DIET or have been following one for years, you can't help but interact with others concerning your choices. Family members or friends may be supportive, or not. As with any dietary approach, there's an abundance of conflicting information you may have to sort through. Here are our suggestions for implementing success strategies to help you navigate the influences that help and those that hinder.

## The Flexible Approach

I've found that flexibility in thinking is one of the most important strategies that I've employed in my approach to raw food. In addition, I've found that being open minded has allowed me to think more critically about my dietary results and enabled me to make changes when necessary.

Sometimes people view dietary approaches as all-or-nothing or tend to idealize one approach as being the ultimate goal. If they have a hard time reaching this ideal, they may get discouraged, fall back into old habits, and not take advantage of intermediate steps to reach that goal. Making small but meaningful changes may be all that someone needs to do, and there's no need to feel unnecessarily pressured. Many people experience health benefits just by making minor changes to their diet, such as eliminating commercially processed or packaged foods and focusing their diet on whole foods.

For many reasons, one person's perfect diet may not be ideal for everyone. It's important to not see a raw food diet as an all-or-nothing proposition. Healthy diets can exist on a spectrum of approaches that are tailored to individual needs. Most of the successful long-term raw-food enthusiasts I've known have made changes to their approaches to suit their evolving needs.

Some people may do better making numerous changes or one large change all at once, while others do best with incremental change, so it's important to keep an open mind about the format and speed in which changes need to be implemented. On the other hand, if someone makes significant changes but still maintains a few habits that don't support health, they may not get the results they're looking for and blame their diet for their shortcoming. At that point, we try to find the reason or reasons for the person's challenge, make changes, and observe the outcome. Future additional changes may also be necessary. I've found that finding dietary balance for someone can often be a work in progress.

## Getting Friends and Family Interested in Healthy Eating

If you really want to get loved ones on board with healthy eating, take it slowly and see how receptive they are to your message. It goes without saying that it's best to not make anyone feel wrong for doing what they're doing; it can create a barrier to communication. Always leave the door open for people who may not be interested in your message at the time, because they may very well be more curious in the future.

When I started eating a raw, plant-based diet, my parents weren't particularly receptive to what I had to say. However, when my mom passed away, my dad was faced with preparing his own food, and he asked me to teach him how to make easy, nutritious dishes that were tasty and appealing. After more than twenty years of observing my dietary choices, he finally became motivated to prepare his own healthy food. Now my dad loves steamed vegetables, salads, green smoothies, and much more. He's noted that both his energy and memory have improved, and he couldn't be happier. He walks and exercises regularly and is able to do all the activities he wants to accomplish. At 89 years old, this means everything to him and I am happy to be in support of his healthy endeavors.

When I began my raw journey, some members of my family were concerned initially with my well-being, which is understandable given that they wanted to make sure that I was doing something safe and beneficial. I explained to them the rationale for this approach to health and the benefits I had experienced from the changes I made. They did agree with me that my increased energy was noticeable, so they were willing to continue the conversation. I explained that I had given this change much thought and research and was happy with the result. I also mentioned that I was remaining open minded to other approaches if a need for change presented itself down the road, and knowing I was flexible helped to put my family at ease. Let family members see that you're happy and healthy. They may even follow your lead if you get the results that they are seeking.

## Sorting Raw-Food Fact from Fiction

Many of our students and people with whom we have spoken over the years have expressed frustration with the seemingly conflicting information about raw foods in particular and alternative health in general. How can so many experts disagree? From my experience, I've seen that sometimes a particular health topic has not been well studied, so we have to rely on clinical experience, personal experience, or both. Or if a topic has been well studied, the clinical answer has yet to become the standard of care. Other times, the success of a particular health program is incorrectly attributed to one reason, or different approaches may actually work well in different situations. In addition, information on a particular health topic may be available, but is unknown, incompletely understood, or misinterpreted by the person speaking or writing.

One of the caveats to consider is sources of raw-food information that are tied in with the sale of products. Sometimes this information is reliable and sometimes it's not. Many products are of excellent quality, useful, and well worth the money, but just because someone said that a product is good does not make it so. Product-based information can also ignore important aspects of health, make eating a raw food diet seem more complicated than it needs to be, or take people down a path that's not in their best health or financial interest. All this information needs to be examined with a critical eye and not just accepted at face value. Here are some questions to ask:

- What is the source of the information?
- Is there a financial interest behind it?
- Is it biased or pushing an agenda?

Look for sources of information that are as unbiased as possible. Choose many reliable sources (including those that challenge your point of view) and seek out rational, reasonable, and evidence-based opinions. If you only expose yourself to information that supports your current thinking, you'll likely find evidence for it, which further reinforces your beliefs (called confirmation bias). Realize that nobody has all the answers; you may need to seek information from multiple sources or practitioners. Be particularly cautious about information that's presented from a negative or sensational perspective. Just because someone says that information is scientifically based does not make it so; do your homework and fact check often. If you can, speak to clinicians, people who can evaluate what you're finding out on the basis of their clinical experience.

Take responsibility for your own health decisions. Be well educated about your health care options. I'm in favor of employing a health care team or a group of health care professionals who have knowledge and skill in the particular area of health care I seek; different providers will have a variety of clinical experiences and educational backgrounds.

In the twenty-five plus years I've spent in the health sciences field, I've learned a tremendous amount and am consistently in awe of how much information is actually available. What's even more exciting is what will be studied in years to come. Research in the field of nutrition (clinical, experimental, and otherwise) is very important, but I also feel that personal experience is equally important. Personal experience or anecdotal evidence may often precede what has been officially researched and can sometimes serve as inspiration for researchers to study certain topics or phenomena. The two can work together, hand in hand, in some cases. There's a lot that we know and a lot more that we have yet to learn.

# Conclusion

⸻∞⸻

THIS BOOK IS JUST A BEGINNING! What you've read here is just a sampling of what I've learned since I became interested in raw food and health in 1990. I hope that what I've shared here has been useful to you. I encourage you to educate yourself about health and add this education to your understanding of health and nutrition.

Food is just one aspect of health, and there are many topics related to personal health that may be of interest to you, such as sustainable agriculture, organic farming, permaculture, animal treatment in agriculture, and more. Understanding these subjects can help us see that we're part of a larger whole, that our actions can have an influence on the world around us, and that our personal health can be influenced by the health of the planet. We cover some of these topics and many others in our Science of Raw Food Nutrition classes, and so I invite you to join us! In the meantime, I wish you the best in your health adventures and encourage you to keep learning. After all, health is much like life—it's more of a journey than a destination.

# Appendix

—∞∞∞—

## Helpful Conversion Factors

- One gram (g) = 1,000 milligrams (mg)
- One milligram (mg) = 1,000 micrograms (mcg or µg)
- One gram (g) = 1,000,000 micrograms (mcg or µg)
- One gram (g) = 0.035 ounces (oz)
- One ounce (oz) = 28.35 g
- One pound (lb) = 454 g = 0.454 kg
- °C = [(°F-32) x 5]/9
- °F = [(°C x 9)/5] + 32

# Resources

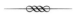

### Nutrient Content of Foods

Food Processor Nutrition and Fitness Software, ESHA Research, Inc. esha.com

USDA National Nutrient Database for Standard Reference. nal.usda.gov/fnic/foodcomp/search/

### General Information on Nutrition and Nutrition Science

Gartner LP, Hiatt JI. *Color Textbook of Histology.* Philadelphia, PA: W.B. Saunders Company, 1997.

Groff JL and Gropper SS. *Advanced Nutrition and Human Metabolism,* 3rd Edition. Belmont, CA: Wadsworth Thomson Learning, 2000.

Guyton, AC. *Textbook of Medical Physiology,* 8th Edition. Philadelphia, PA: W.B. Saunders Company, 1991.

Masterton WL, Hurley CN, Neth EJ. *Chemistry: Principles and Reactions,* Seventh Edition. Belmont, CA. Brooks/Cole, Cengage Learning, 2012.

Raven PH, Evert RF, Eichhorn SE. *Biology of Plants,* 7th Edition. New York: W.H. Freeman and Company, 2005.

Salway J. *Metabolism at a Glance,* 2nd Edition. Malden, MA: Blackwell Science Ltd, 1999.

Zomlefer W. *Guide to Flowering Plant Families.* Chapel Hill, North Carolina: The University of North Carolina Press, 1994.

Zubay GL. *Biochemistry,* Fourth Edition. Dubuque, IA: Wm C. Brown Publishers, 1998.

### Dietary Reference Intakes (DRIs), including Adequate Intakes (AIs) and Recommended Dietary Allowances (RDAs)

"Dietary Guidelines." US Department of Health and Human Services, The Office of Disease Prevention and Health Promotion. dietaryguidelines.gov

Dietary Reference Intakes. National Academy of Sciences, Institute of Medicine, Food and Nutrition Board. fnic.nal.usda.gov/dietary-guidance/dietary-reference-intakes/dri-tables

Food and Nutrition Board, Institute of Medicine. *Dietary Reference Intakes for Thiamin, Riboflavin, Niacin, Vitamin B$_6$, Folate, Pantothenic Acid, Biotin, and Choline.* Washington, DC: National Academy Press, 1998.

Institute of Medicine of the National Academies, Food and Nutrition Board. *Dietary Reference Intakes for Energy, Carbohydrate, Fiber, Fat, Fatty Acids, Cholesterol, Protein, and Amino Acids (Macronutrients).* Washington, DC: National Academies Press, 2005.

National Academy of Sciences, Institute of Medicine, Food and Nutrition Board. *Dietary Reference Intakes for Vitamin A, Vitamin K, Arsenic, Boron, Chromium, Copper, Iodine, Iron, Manganese, Molybdenum, Nickel, Silicon, Vanadium, and Zinc.* (2001)

_____ "Vitamin A." nal.usda.gov/fnic/DRI//DRI_Vitamin_A/82-161_150.pdf

U.S. Department of Agriculture and U.S. Department of Health and Human Services. *Dietary Guidelines for Americans, 2010.* 7th Edition, Washington, DC: U.S. Government Printing Office, December 2010.

# References

## Chapter 1: What Is Raw?

Azocar J, Diaz A. Efficacy and safety of Chlorella supplementation in adults with chronic hepatitis C virus infection. *World J Gastroenterol*. 2013 Feb 21;19(7):1085–90.

Brenes M, García A, Dobarganes MC, Velasco J, Romero C. Influence of thermal treatments simulating cooking processes on the polyphenol content in virgin olive oil. *J Agric Food Chem*. 2002 Oct 9;50(21):5962–7.

Ginde AA, Liu MC, Camargo CA Jr. Demographic differences and trends of vitamin D insufficiency in the US population, 1988–2004. *Arch Intern Med*. 2009 Mar 23;169(6):626–32.

Gómez-Alonso S, Fregapane G, Salvador MD, Gordon MH. Changes in phenolic composition and antioxidant activity of virgin olive oil during frying. *J Agric Food Chem*. 2003 Jan 29;51(3):667–72.

González-Rodríguez LG, Estaire P, Peñas-Ruiz C, Ortega RM. Vitamin D intake and dietary sources in a representative sample of Spanish adults. *J Hum Nutr Diet*. 2013 Apr 19.

Hendler S, Rorvik D. *PDR for Nutritional Supplements*, Second Edition. Montvale, NJ: Physician's Desk Reference Inc., 2008.

John S, Sorokin AV, Thompson PD. Phytosterols and vascular disease. *Curr Opin Lipidol*. 2007 Feb;18(1):35–40.

Juntunen KS, Niskanen LK, Liukkonen KH, Poutanen KS, Holst JJ, Mykkänen HM. Postprandial glucose, insulin, and incretin responses to grain products in healthy subjects. *Am J Clin Nutr*. 2002 Feb;75(2):254–62.

Kang J, Weylandt K. Modulation of inflammatory cytokines by omega-3 fatty acids. *Subcell Biochem*. 2008;49:133–43.

Link LB, Jacobson JS. Factors affecting adherence to a raw vegan diet. *Complement Ther Clin Pract*. 2008 Feb;14(1):53–9.

Lowe MR, Tappe KA, Butryn ML, et al. An intervention study targeting energy and nutrient intake in worksite cafeterias. *Eat Behav*. 2010 Aug;11(3):144–51.

Mozaffarian D. Trans fatty acids – effects on systemic inflammation and endothelial function. *Atheroscler Suppl*. 2006;7(2):29–32.

Mozaffarian D, Willett W. Trans fatty acids and cardiovascular risk: a unique cardiometabolic imprint? *Curr Atheroscler Rep*. 2007;9(6):486–93.

Murphy MM, Barraj LM, Herman D, Bi X, Cheatham R, Randolph RK. Phytonutrient Intake by Adults in the United States in Relation to Fruit and Vegetable Consumption. *J Am Diet Assoc*. 2011 Nov 9.

Resnik D. Trans fat bans and human freedom. *Am J Bioeth*. 2010 Mar;10(3):27–32.

Rolls BJ, Drewnowski A, Ledikwe JH. Changing the energy density of the diet as a strategy for weight management. *J Am Diet Assoc*. 2005 May;105(5 Suppl 1):S98–103.

Shytle DR, Tan J, Ehrhart J, et al. Effects of blue-green algae extracts on the proliferation of human adult stem cells in vitro: a preliminary study. *Med Sci Monit*. 2010 Jan;16(1):BR1–5.

Simopoulos AP. The importance of the ratio of omega-6/omega-3 essential fatty acids. *Biomed Pharmacother*. 2002;56(8):365–79.

Sommer A, Vyas KS. A global clinical view on vitamin A and carotenoids. *Am J Clin Nutr*. 2012 Nov;96(5):1204S–6S.

Song JH, Fujimoto K, Miyazawa T. Polyunsaturated (n-3) fatty acids susceptible to peroxidation are increased in plasma and tissue lipids of rats fed docosahexaenoic acid-containing oils. *J Nutr*. 2000 Dec;130(12):3028–33.

Tucker K. Hannan M, Kiel D. The acid-base hypothesis: diet and bone in the Framingham Osteoporosis study. *Eur J Nutr.* 2001;40(5):231–7.

Verhaeghe EF, Fraysse A, Guerquin-Kern JL, et al. Microchemical imaging of iodine distribution in the brown alga Laminaria digitata suggests a new mechanism for its accumulation. *J Biol Inorg Chem.* 2008 Feb;13(2):257–69.

Yetley EA. Assessing the vitamin D status of the US population. *Am J Clin Nutr.* 2008 Aug;88(2):558S–564S.

Yuan YV, Carrington MF, Walsh NA. Extracts from dulse (Palmaria palmata) are effective antioxidants and inhibitors of cell proliferation in vitro. *Food Chem Toxicol.* 2005 Jul;43(7):1073–81.

## Chapter 2: Carbohydrates and Fiber

Alkaabi JM, Al-Dabbagh B, Ahmad S, Saadi HF, Gariballa S, Ghazali MA. Glycemic indices of five varieties of dates in healthy and diabetic subjects. *Nutr J.* 2011 May 28;10:59.

Atkinson F, Foster-Powell K, Brand-Miller J. International tables of glycemic index and glycemic load values: 2008. *Diabetes Care.* 2008;31(12):2281–3.

Berg JM, Tymoczko JL, Stryer L. *Biochemistry.* 5th edition. New York: W H Freeman; 2002.

Bocarsly M, Powell E, Avena N, Hoebel B. High-fructose corn syrup causes characteristics of obesity in rats: Increased body weight, body fat and triglyceride levels. *Pharmacol Biochem Behav.* 2010 Feb 26. [Epub ahead of print]

Campbell J, Bauer L, Fahey G, Hogarth A, Wolf B, Hunter D. Selected Fructooligosaccharide (1-Kestose, Nystose, and 1$^F$--Fructofuranosylnystose) Composition of Foods and Feeds. *J. Agric. Food Chem.* 1997;45(8):3076–3082.

Foster-Powell K, Holt S, Brand-Miller J. International table of glycemic index and glycemic load values: 2002. *Am J Clin Nutr.* 2002;76(1):5–56.

Freudenheim JL, Marshall JR, Vena JE, et al. Premenopausal breast cancer risk and intake of vegetables, fruits, and related nutrients. *J Natl Cancer Inst.* 1996 Mar 20;88(6):340–8.

Fulgoni V. High-fructose corn syrup: everything you wanted to know, but were afraid to ask. *Am J Clin Nutr.* 2008;88(6):1715S.

Hijova E, Chmelarova A. Short chain fatty acids and colonic health. *Bratisl Lek Listy.* 2007;108(8):354-358.

Holt SH, Miller JC, Petocz P. An insulin index of foods: the insulin demand generated by 1000-kJ portions of common foods. *Am J Clin Nutr.* 1997 Nov;66(5):1264–76.

Kelly G. Inulin-type prebiotics–a review: part 1. *Altern Med Rev.* 2008 Dec;13(4):315–29.

Komatsu T, Shoji N, Saito K, Suzuki K. Effects of genetic and environmental factors on muscle glycogen content in Japanese Black cattle. *Anim Sci J.* 2014 Aug;85(8):793-8

Lau DC, Douketis JD, Morrison KM, Hramiak IM, Sharma AM, Ur E; Obesity Canada Clinical Practice Guidelines Expert Panel. 2006 Canadian clinical practice guidelines on the management and prevention of obesity in adults and children [summary]. *CMAJ.* 2007;176(8):S1–13.

Leach JD, Sobolik KD. High dietary intake of prebiotic inulin-type fructans in the prehistoric Chihuahuan Desert. *Br J Nutr.* 2010 Jun;103(11):1558–61.

Livesey G. Health potential of polyols as sugar replacers, with emphasis on low glycaemic properties. *Nutr Res Rev.* 2003 Dec;16(2):163–91.

Miller C, Dunn E, Hashim I. Glycemic index of 3 varieties of dates. *Saudi Med J.* 2002;23(5):536–8.

Niness K. Inulin and oligofructose: what are they? *J Nutr* 1999; 129 (7 Suppl): 1402S–1406S.

Van Loo J, Coussement P, de Leenheer L, Hoebregs H, Smits G. On the presence of inulin and oligofructose as natural ingredients in the western diet. *Crit Rev Food Sci Nutr.* 1995;35(6):525–52.

Wong JM, de Souza R, Kendall CW, Emam A, Jenkins DJ. Colonic health: fermentation and short chain fatty acids. *J Clin Gastroenterol.* 2006 Mar;40(3):235–43.

## Chapter 3: Fat

Akanda MJ, Sarker MZ, Ferdosh S, Manap MY, Ab Rahman NN, Ab Kadir MO. Applications of supercritical fluid extraction (SFE) of palm oil and oil from natural sources. *Molecules.* 2012 Feb 10;17(2):1764–94.

Carlson SJ, Fallon EM, Kalish BT, Gura KM, Puder M. The role of the omega-3 fatty acid DHA in the human life cycle. *J Parenter Enteral Nutr.* 2013 Jan;37(1):15–22.

Chakrabarty MM. *Chemistry and Technology of Oils and Fats.* Mumbai, India: Allied Publishers Pvt. Limited, 2003.

Choi JK, Ho J, Curry S, Qin D, Bittman R, Hamilton JA. Interactions of very long-chain saturated fatty acids with serum albumin. *J Lipid Res.* 2002 Jul;43(7):1000–10.

Conquer JA, Holub BJ. Supplementation with an algae source of docosahexaenoic acid increases (n-3) fatty acid status and alters selected risk factors for heart disease in vegetarian subjects. *J Nutr.* 1996 Dec;126(12):3032–9.

European Food Safety Authority. Scientific Opinion on the Tolerable Upper Intake Level of Eicosapentaenoic Acid (EPA), Docosahexaenoic Acid (DHA), and Docosapentaenoic Acid (DPA). 2012. efsa. europa.eu/en/efsajournal/doc/2815.pdf

Fanali C, Dugo L, Cacciola F, et al. Chemical characterization of Sacha Inchi (Plukenetia volubilis L.) oil. *J Agric Food Chem.* 2011;59(24): 13043–9. doi: 10.1021/jf203184y.

Follegatti-Romero L, Piantino C, Grimaldi R, Cabral F. Supercritical $CO_2$ extraction of omega-3 rich oil from Sacha Inchi (Plukenetia volubilis L.) seeds. *The Journal of Supercritical Fluids* 2009;49(3):323–329.

Greenberg JA, Bell SJ, Ausdal WV. Omega-3 Fatty Acid supplementation during pregnancy. *Rev Obstet Gynecol.* 2008 Fall;1(4):162–9.

Hamaker B, Valles C, Gilman R, et al. Amino acid and fatty acid profiles of the Inca Peanut (Plukenetia volubilis L.). *Cereal Chemistry* 1992;6(4):461–463.

Hu FB, Stampfer MJ, Manson JE, et al. Dietary saturated fats and their food sources in relation to the risk of coronary heart disease in women. *Am J Clin Nutr.* 1999 Dec;70(6):1001–8.

Huang CB, Alimova Y, Myers TM, Ebersole JL. Short- and medium-chain fatty acids exhibit antimicrobial activity for oral microorganisms. *Arch Oral Biol.* 2011 Jul;56(7):650–4.

Knothe G, Dunn RO. A comprehensive evaluation of the melting points of fatty acids and esters determined by differential scanning calorimetry. *J Am Oil Chem Soc.* 2009;86:843–856.

Layden BT, Angueira AR, Brodsky M, Durai V, Lowe WL Jr. Short chain fatty acids and their receptors: new metabolic targets. *Transl Res.* 2013 Mar;161(3):131–40.

Lenihan-Geels G, Bishop KS, Ferguson LR. Alternative sources of omega-3 fats: can we find a sustainable substitute for fish? *Nutrients.* 2013 Apr 18;5(4):1301–15.

Lovegren NV, Gray MS, Feuge RO. Effect of liquid fat on melting point and polymorphic behavior of cocoa butter and a cocoa butter fraction. *Journal of the American Oil Chemists Society.* 1976;53(3):108–112.

Maurer N, Hatta-Sakoda B, Pascual-Chagman G, Rodriguez-Saona L. Characterization and authentication of a novel vegetable source of omega-3 fatty acids, sacha inchi (Plukenetia volubilis L.) oil. *Food Chemistry.* 2012;134:1173–1180.

Metcalf JH, Donoghue AM, Venkitanarayanan K, et al. Water administration of the medium-chain fatty acid caprylic acid produced variable efficacy against enteric Campylobacter colonization in broilers. *Poult Sci.* 2011 Feb;90(2):494–7.

Mozaffarian D. Does alpha-linolenic acid intake reduce the risk of coronary heart disease? A review of the evidence. *Altern Ther Health Med.* 2005 May-Jun;11(3):24–30; quiz 31, 79.

Rego Costa AC, Rosado EL, Soares-Mota M. Influence of the dietary intake of medium chain triglycerides on body composition, energy expenditure and satiety: a systematic review. *Nutr Hosp.* 2012 Jan-Feb;27(1):103–8.

St. Onge MP, Bosarge A, Goree LL, Darnell B. Medium chain triglyceride oil consumption as part of a weight loss diet does not lead to an adverse metabolic profile when compared to olive oil. *J Am Coll Nutr.* 2008; 27(5):547–552.

Schwalfenberg G. Omega-3 fatty acids: their beneficial role in cardiovascular health. *Canadian Family Physician* 2006;52:734–740.

Seaton TB, Welle SL, Warenko MK, Campbell RG. Thermic effect of medium-chain and long-chain triglycerides in man. *Am J Clin Nutr.* 1986 Nov;44(5):630–4.

Simopoulos AP. The importance of the ratio of omega-6/omega-3 essential fatty acids. *Biomed Pharmacother.* 2002;56(8):365–79.

Simopoulos AP. Omega-3/Omega-6 essential fatty acid ratio and chronic diseases. *Food Reviews International.* 2004;20(1):77–90.

Simopoulos AP. The importance of the omega-6/omega-3 fatty acid ratio in cardiovascular disease and other chronic diseases. *Exp Biol Med (Maywood).* 2008 Jun;233(6):674–88.

Song JH, Fujimoto K, Miyazawa T. Polyunsaturated (n-3) fatty acids susceptible to peroxidation are increased in plasma and tissue lipids of rats fed docosahexaenoic acid-containing oils. *J Nutr.* 2000 Dec;130(12):3028–33.

Sonwai S, Ponprachanuvut P. Characterization of physicochemical and thermal properties and crystallization behavior of krabok (irvingia malayana) and rambutan seed fats. *J Oleo Sci.* 2012;61(12):671–9.

## Chapter 4: Protein

Azara CR, Maia IC, Rangel CN, et al. Ethanol Intake during Lactation Alters Milk Nutrient Composition and Growth and Mineral Status of Rat Pups. *Biol Res.* 2008;41(3):317–330. p.323, table 2.

Birlouez-Aragon I, Leclere J, Quedraogo CL, Birlouez E, Grongnet JF. The FAST method, a rapid approach of the nutritional quality of heat-treated foods. *Nahrung.* 2001;45(3):201-5.

Carter HE, Coon MJ. *Biographical Memoir for William Cumming Rose*, Vol. 68. Washington, DC: National Academy of Sciences, 1995.

Cho ES, Anderson HL, Wixom RL, Hanson KC, Krause GF. Long-term effects of low histidine intake on men. *Journal of Nutrition*, 1984, 114:369–384.

da Rocha EE, Alves VG, Silva MH, Chiesa CA, da Fonseca RB. Can measured resting energy expenditure be estimated by formulae in daily clinical nutrition practice? *Curr Opin Clin Nutr Metab Care.* 2005 May;8(3):319–28.

Davis TA, Nguyen HV, Garcia-Bravo R, et al. Amino Acid Composition of Human Milk is Not Unique. *J. Nutr.* 1994;124:1126-1132.

Drouin G, Godin JR, Pagé B. The genetics of vitamin C loss in vertebrates. *Curr Genomics.* 2011 Aug;12(5):371–8.

Dworschák E. Nonenzyme browning and its effect on protein nutrition. *Crit Rev Food Sci Nutr.* 1980;13(1):1–40.

Ensminger A, Ensminger M, Konlade J, Robson J. *Foods and Nutrition Encyclopedia*, Second Edition, Volume II. Boca Raton, FL: CRC-Press, 1993.

Erbersdobler HF, Hupe A. Determination of lysine damage and calculation of lysine bio-availability in several processed foods. *Z Ernahrungswiss*. 1991;30(1):46–9

Furst P. Stehle P. What are the essential elements needed for the determination of amino acid requirements in humans? *J Nutr*. 2004;134(6):1558S–1565S.

Hurrell RF, Finot, PA. Food processing and storage as a determinant of protein and amino acid availability. *Experientia Suppl*. 1983;44:135–56.

Jenness R. The composition of human milk. *Semin Perinatol*. 1979;3(3):225–39.

Kopple JD, Swendseid ME. Evidence that histidine is an essential amino acid in normal and chronically uremic man. *Journal of Clinical Investigation*. 1975;55:881–891.

Kopple JD, Swendseid ME. Effect of histidine intake on plasma and urine histidine levels, nitrogen balance and N-tau-methylhistidine excretion in normal and chronically uremic men. *Journal of Nutrition*. 1981;111:931–942.

Mauron J. Influence of processing on protein quality. *J Nutr Sci Vitaminol* (Tokyo). 1990;36 Suppl 1:S57–69.

Nakagawa I, Takahashi T, Suzuki T, Kobayashi K. Amino acid requirements of children: minimal needs for tryptophan, arginine and histidine based on nitrogen balance method. *Journal of Nutrition*, 1963, 80:305–308.

Pellett PL. Food energy requirements in humans. *Am J Clin Nutr*. 1990 May;51(5):711–22.

Pizzoferrato L, Manzi P, Vivanti V, Nicoletti I, Corradini C, Cogliandro E. Maillard reaction in mild-based foods: nutritional consequences. *J Food Prot*. 1998;61(2):235-9.

Reeds PJ. Dispensable and indispensable amino acids for humans. *J Nutr*. 2000;130(7):1835S–1840S.

Roe D. William Cumming Rose: A Biographical Sketch. *J. Nutr.* 1981;111:1311–1320.

Rose W. The sequence of events leading to the establishment of the amino acid needs of man. *Am J Publ Health*. 1968;58(11):2020–7.

Roza AM, Shizgal HM. The Harris Benedict equation reevaluated: resting energy requirements and the body cell mass. *Am J Clin Nutr*. 1984 Jul;40(1):168–82.

Simoni RD, Hill RL, Vaughan M. Nutritional Biochemistry and the Amino Acid Composition of Proteins: the Early Years of Protein Chemistry. The Work of Thomas B. Osborne and Lafayette B. Mendel. *J Biol Chem*. 2002;277(18):E7.

Simoni R, Hill R, Vaughan M. The discovery of the amino acid threonine: the work of William C. Rose. *J Biol Chem* 2002;277(37):E25.

Wixom RL, Anderson HL, Terry BE, Sheng YB. Total parenteral nutrition with selective histidine depletion in man. I. Responses in nitrogen metabolism and related areas. *American Journal of Clinical Nutrition*. 1977;30(6):887–899.

World Health Organization. *Protein and Amino Acid Requirements in Human Nutrition*. Geneva, Switzerland: WHO Press, 2007.

## Chapter 5: Minerals

Afify Ael-M, El-Beltagi HS, El-Salam SM, Omran AA. Bioavailability of iron, zinc, phytate and phytase activity during soaking and germination of white sorghum varieties. *PLoS One*. 2011;6(10):e25512.

Alissa EM, Bahijri SM, Ferns GA. The controversy surrounding selenium and cardiovascular disease: a review of the evidence. *Med Sci Monit*. 2003 Jan;9(1):RA9–18.

Beckett G, Nicol F, Rae P, Beech S, Guo Y, Arthur J. Effects of combined iodine and selenium deficiency on thyroid hormone metabolism in rats. *Am J Clin Nutr*. 1993;57(2 Suppl):240S–243S.

Bohn L, Meyer AS, Rasmussen SK. Phytate: impact on environment and human nutrition. A challenge for molecular breeding. *J Zhejiang Univ Sci B*. 2008 Mar;9(3):165–91. doi: 10.1631/jzus.B0710640.

Chai W, Liebman M. Effect of different cooking methods on vegetable oxalate content. *J Agric Food Chem*. 2005;53(8):3027–30.

Cook J, Reddy M. Effect of ascorbic acid intake on non-heme iron absorption from a complete diet. *Am J Clin Nutr* 2001;73:93–8.

Darling AL, Millward DJ, Torgerson DJ, Hewitt CE, Lanham-New SA. Dietary protein and bone health: a systematic review and meta-analysis. *Am J Clin Nutr*. 2009;90(6):1674–92.

Etcheverry P, Grusak MA, Fleige LE. Application of in vitro bioaccessibility and bioavailability methods for calcium, carotenoids, folate, iron, magnesium, polyphenols, zinc, and vitamins B(6), B(12), D, and E. *Front Physiol*. 2012;3:317.

Ferruzzi M, Blakesleeb J. Digestion, absorption, and cancer preventative activity of dietary chlorophyll derivatives. *Nutrition Research* 2007;27(1):1–12.

Ferruzzi M, Failla M, Schwartz S. Assessment of degradation and intestinal cell uptake of carotenoids and chlorophyll derivatives from spinach puree using an in vitro digestion and Caco-2 human cell model. *J Agric Food Chem*. 2001 Apr;49(4):2082–9.

Frazer D, Anderson G. Iron imports. I. Intestinal iron absorption and its regulation. *Am J Physiol Gastrointest Liver Physiol* 2005;289:G631–G635

Gibson RS, Perlas L, Hotz C. Improving the bioavailability of nutrients in plant foods at the household level. *Proc Nutr Soc*. 2006 May;65(2):160–8.

Holick M. Sunlight and vitamin D for bone health and prevention of autoimmune diseases, cancers, and cardiovascular disease. *Am J Clin Nutr*. 2004 Dec;80(6 Suppl):1678S–88S.

Holick MF, Biancuzzo RM, Chen TC, et al. Vitamin D2 is as effective as vitamin D3 in maintaining circulating concentrations of 25-hydroxyvitamin D. *J Clin Endocrinol Metab*. 2008 Mar;93(3):677–81.

Holmes RP, Kennedy M. Estimation of the oxalate content of foods and daily oxalate intake. *Kidney Int*. 2000 Apr;57(4):1662–7.

Hotz C, Gibson RS. Traditional food-processing and preparation practices to enhance the bioavailability of micronutrients in plant-based diets. *J Nutr*. 2007 Apr;137(4):1097–100.

Hunt J. Bioavailability of iron, zinc, and other trace minerals from vegetarian diets. *Am J Clin Nutr* 2003;78(suppl):633S–9S.

Hunt J. High-, but not low-bioavailability diets enable substantial control of women's iron absorption in relation to body iron stores, with minimal adaptation within several weeks. *Am J Clin Nutr* 2003;78:1168–77.

Hunt J, Roughead Z. Adaptation of iron absorption in men consuming diets with high or low iron bioavailability. *Am J Clin Nutr* 2000;71:94–102.

Hurrell R, Egli I. Iron bioavailability and dietary reference values. *Am J Clin Nutr* 2010;91(suppl):1461S–7S.

Lanham-New S. The balance of bone health: tipping the scales in favor of potassium-rich, bicarbonate-rich foods. *J Nutr*. 2008;138(1):172S–177S.

Lin PH, Ginty F, Appel LJ, et al. The DASH diet and sodium reduction improve markers of bone turnover and calcium metabolism in adults. *J Nutr*. 2003;133(10):3130–6.

Macfarlane BJ, Bezwoda WR, Bothwell TH, et al. Inhibitory effect of nuts on iron absorption. *Am J Clin Nutr*. 1988 Feb;47(2):270–4.

Mate H, Radomir L. Phytic acid content of cereals and legumes and interaction with proteins. *Periodica Polytechnica Ser. Chem. Eng*. 2002;46(1-2):59–64.

Morton Salt, Inc. Morton table salt and sea salt labels. mortonsalt.com/for-your-home/culinary-salts/food-salts/19/morton-all-purpose-sea-salt.

_____mortonsalt.com/for-your-home/culinary-salts/food-salts/1/morton-table-salt-plain-and-iodized/

New SA. Nutrition Society Medal lecture. The role of the skeleton in acid-base homeostasis. *Proc Nutr Soc.* 2002 May;61(2):151–64.

New SA. Intake of fruit and vegetables: implications for bone health. *Proc Nutr Soc.* 2003 Nov;62(4):889–99.

New SA and Millward DJ. Calcium, protein, fruit, and vegetables as dietary determinants of bone health. *Am J of Clinical Nutrition.* 2003;77(5):1340–1341.

New SA, Robins SP, Campbell MK, et al. Dietary influences on bone mass and bone metabolism: further evidence of a positive link between fruit and vegetable consumption and bone health? *Am J Clin Nutr.* 2000;71(1):142–51.

Nielsen F. How should dietary guidance be given for mineral elements with beneficial actions or suspected of being essential? *J Nutr.* 1996;126(9 Suppl):2377S–2385S.

Nimni M, Han B, Cordoba F. Are we getting enough sulfur in our diet? *Nutrition and Metabolism.* 2007 Nov 6;4(24).

Noonan SC, Savage GP. Oxalate content of foods and its effect on humans. *Asia Pacific J Clin Nutr* 1999;8(1):64–74.

Reddy NR, Sathe SK. *Food Phytates.* Boca Raton, FL. CRC Press, LLC, 2001.

Remer T. Influence of diet on acid-base balance. *Semin Dial.* 2000;13(4):221–6.

Remer T, Manz F. Potential renal acid load of foods and its influence on urine pH. *J Am Diet Assoc.* 1995;95(7):791–7.

Rickard A, Chatfield M, Conway R, Stephen A, Powell J. An algorithm to assess intestinal iron availability for use in dietary surveys. *Br J Nutr* 2009;102(11):1678–1685.

Sakhaee K. Recent advances in the pathophysiology of nephrolithiasis. *Kidney Int.* 2009 Mar;75(6):585-95.

Sandberg AS. Bioavailability of minerals in legumes. *Br J Nutr.* 2002;88 Suppl 3:S281–5.

Sandberg AS. The effect of food processing on phytate hydrolysis and availability of iron and zinc. *Adv Exp Med Biol.* 1991;289:499–508.

Schwalfenberg GK. The alkaline diet: is there evidence that an alkaline pH diet benefits health? *J Environ Public Health.* 2012;2012:727630. Epub 2011 Oct 12.

Sebastian A, Frassetto LA, Sellmeyer DE, Merriam RL, Morris RC Jr. Estimation of the net acid load of the diet of ancestral preagricultural Homo sapiens and their hominid ancestors. *Am J Clin Nutr.* 2002;76(6):1308–16.

Tucker K, Hannan M, Chen H, Cupples L, Wilson P, Kiel D. Potassium, magnesium, and fruit and vegetable intakes are associated with greater bone mineral density in elderly men and women. *Am J Clin Nutr.* 1999;69(4):727–36.

Tucker K. Hannan M, Kiel D. The acid-base hypothesis: diet and bone in the Framingham Osteoporosis study. *Eur J Nutr.* 2001;40(5):231–7.

US Department of Agriculture, Agricultural Research Service. "Oxalic Acid Content of Selected Vegetables." ars.usda.gov/Services/docs.htm?docid=9444.

Weaver CM, Heaney RP. *Calcium in Human Health.* Totowa, NJ. W.B. Humana Press, 2006.

Weaver CM, Heaney RP, Nickel KP, Packard PI. Calcium Bioavailability from high oxalate vegetables: Chinese vegetables, sweet potatoes, and rhubarb. *J Food Sci.* 1997;62:524–5.

Weaver CM, Liebman M. Biomarkers of bone health appropriate for evaluating functional foods designed to reduce risk of osteoporosis. *Br J Nutr.* 2002;88 Suppl 2:S225–32.

Weaver CM, Proulx WR, Heaney RP. Choices for achieving adequate dietary calcium with a vegetarian diet. *American Journal of Clinical Nutrition.* 1999;70(suppl):543S–8S.

Welch A, Mulligan A, Bingham S, Khaw K. Urine pH is an indicator of dietary acid-base load, fruit and vegetables and meat intakes: results from the European Prospective Investigation into Cancer and Nutrition (EPIC) – Norfolk population study. *Br J Nutr.* 2008;99(6):1335–43.

Whiting S, Muirhead J. Measurement of net acid excretion by use of paper strips. *Nutrition.* 2005;21(9):961–3.

Yanatori I, Tabuchi M, Kawai Y, Yasui Y, Akagi R, Kishi F. Heme and non-heme iron transporters in non-polarized and polarized cells. *BMC Cell Biology.* 2010;11:39.

## Chapter 6: Vitamins

Agarwal S, Rao A. Tomato lycopene and its role in human health and chronic diseases. *CMAJ.* 2000;163(6):739–44.

Albanes, D., Heinonen, O. P., Huttunen, J. K., et al. Effects of alpha-tocopherol and beta-carotene supplements on cancer incidence in the alpha-tocopherol beta-carotene cancer prevention study. *The American Journal of Clinical Nutrition, 62*(6 Suppl), 1427S–1430S.

Alpha-Tocopherol, Beta Carotene Cancer Prevention Study Group. The effect of vitamin E and beta carotene on the incidence of lung cancer and other cancers in male smokers. *N Engl J Med.* 1994;330(15):1029-35.

Barja G. Updating the mitochondrial free radical theory of aging: an integrated view, key aspects and confounding concepts. *Antioxid Redox Signal.* 2013 Oct 20;19(12):1420-45.

Baroni L, Scoglio S, Benedetti S, et al. Effect of a Klamath algae product ("AFA-B$_{12}$") on blood levels of vitamin B$_{12}$ and homocysteine in vegan subjects: a pilot study. *Int J Vitam Nutr Res.* 2009 Mar;79(2):117–23.

Bunyaratavej N. Experience of vitamin K$_2$ in Thailand. *Clin Calcium.* 2007 Nov;17(11):1752–60.

Burri BJ, Clifford AJ. Carotenoid and retinoid metabolism: insights from isotope studies. *Arch Biochem Biophys.* 2004 Oct 1;430(1):110–9.

Cárcamo JM, Pedraza A, Bórquez-Ojeda O, Zhang B, Sanchez R, Golde DW. Vitamin C is a kinase inhibitor: dehydroascorbic acid inhibits IkappaBalpha kinase beta. *Mol Cell Biol.* 2004 Aug;24(15):6645–52.

Castello L, Froio T, Cavallini G, et al. Calorie restriction protects against age-related rat aorta sclerosis. *FASEB J.* 2005 Nov;19(13):1863–5.

Dagnelie PC, van Staveren WA, van den Berg H. Vitamin B-12 from algae appears not to be bioavailable. *Am J Clin Nutr.* 1991;53(3):695–7.

Danoux L, Mine S, Abdul-Malak N, et al. How to help the skin cope with glycoxidation. *Clin Chem Lab Med.* 2013 Apr 2:1–8.

Dib Taxi CM, de Menezes HC, Santos AB, Grosso CR. Study of the microencapsulation of camu-camu (Myrciaria dubia) juice. *J Microencapsul.* 2003 Jul-Aug;20(4):443–8.

Donaldson MS. Metabolic vitamin B$_{12}$ status on a mostly raw vegan diet with follow-up using tablets, nutritional yeast, or probiotic supplements. *Ann Nutr Metab.* 2000;44(5-6):229–34.

Driskell JA, Wollinsky I. *Sports Nutrition: Vitamins and Trace Elements,* Second Edition. Boca Raton, FL: Taylor and Francis Group, 2006.

Du J, Cullen JJ, Buettner GR. Ascorbic acid: chemistry, biology and the treatment of cancer. *Biochim Biophys Acta.* 2012 Dec;1826(2):443–57.

Elmadfa I, Singer I. Vitamin B-12 and homocysteine status among vegetarians: a global perspective. *Am J Clin Nutr.* 2009;89(5):1693S–1698S.

Engelmann NJ, Clinton SK, Erdman JW Jr. Nutritional aspects of phytoene and phytofluene, carotenoid precursors to lycopene. *Adv Nutr.* 2011 Jan;2(1):51–61.

Etminan M, Takkouche B, Caamano-Isorna F. The role of tomato products and lycopene in the prevention of prostate cancer: a meta-analysis of observational studies. *Cancer Epidemiol Biomarkers Prev.* 2004;13(3):340–5.

Fischbach, F. *A Manual of Laboratory and Diagnosic Tests*, Sixth Edition. Philadelphia, PA: Lippincott Williams and Wilkins, 2000.

Fleshman, Matthew Kintz. *Beta Carotene Absorption and Metabolism*. Ph.D. dissertation, Ohio State University, 2011.

Food and Nutrition Board, Institute of Medicine. *Dietary Reference Intakes for Thiamin, Riboflavin, Niacin, Vitamin B6, Folate, Pantothenic Acid, Biotin, and Choline.* Washington, D.C. National Academy Press, 1998.

Hendler S, Rorvik D. *PDR for Nutritional Supplements*, Second Edition. Montvale, NJ: Physician's Desk Reference Inc., 2008.

Ho CC, de Moura FF, Kim SH, Burri BJ, Clifford AJ. A minute dose of 14C-{beta}-carotene is absorbed and converted to retinoids in humans. *J Nutr.* 2009 Aug;139(8):1480–6.

Holick M. Sunlight and vitamin D for bone health and prevention of autoimmune diseases, cancers, and cardiovascular disease. *Am J Clin Nutr.* 2004 Dec;80(6 Suppl):1678S–88S.

Holick M. Vitamin D: extraskeletal health. *Endocrinol Metab Clin North Am.* 2010;39(2):381–400.

Holick MF, Biancuzzo RM, Chen TC, et al. Vitamin $D_2$ is as effective as vitamin $D_3$ in maintaining circulating concentrations of 25-hydroxyvitamin D. *J Clin Endocrinol Metab.* 2008 Mar;93(3):677–81.

Holick MF, Chen TC, Lu Z, Sauter E. Vitamin D and skin physiology: a D-lightful story. *J Bone Miner Res.* 2007 Dec;22 Suppl 2:V28–33.

Justi KC, Visentainer JV, Evelázio de Souza N, Matsushita M. Nutritional composition and vitamin C stability in stored camu-camu (Myrciaria dubia) pulp. *Arch Latinoam Nutr.* 2000 Dec;50(4):405–8.

Khachik F, Carvalho L, Bernstein PS, Muir GJ, Zhao DY, Katz NB. Chemistry, distribution, and metabolism of tomato carotenoids and their impact on human health. *Exp Biol Med* (Maywood). 2002 Nov;227(10):845–51.

Koebnick C, Garcia AL, Dagnelie PC, et al. Long-term consumption of a raw food diet is associated with favorable serum LDL cholesterol and triglycerides but also with elevated plasma homocysteine and low serum HDL cholesterol in humans. *J Nutr.* 2005;135(10):2372–8.

Komai M, Shirakawa H. Vitamin K metabolism. Menaquinone-4 (MK-4) formation from ingested VK analogues and its potent relation to bone function. *Clin Calcium.* 2007 Nov;17(11):1663–72.

Krishnadev N, Meleth AD, Chew EY. Nutritional supplements for age-related macular degeneration. *Curr Opin Ophthalmol.* 2010;21(3):184–9.

Lee HJ, Ju J, Paul S, et al. Mixed tocopherols prevent mammary tumorigenesis by inhibiting estrogen action and activating PPAR-gamma. *Clin Cancer Res.* 2009;15(12):4242–9.

Manzanares W, Hardy G. Vitamin $B_{12}$: the forgotten micronutrient for critical care. *Curr Opin Clin Nutr Metab Care.* 2010 Nov;13(6):662–8.

Matsuoka LY, Ide L, Wortsman J, MacLaughlin J, Holick MF. Sunscreens suppress cutaneous vitamin $D_3$ synthesis. *J Clin Endocrinol Metab.* 1987 64:1165–1168.

Matsuzaki S, Szweda PA, Szweda LI, Humphries KM. Regulated production of free radicals by the mitochondrial electron transport chain: Cardiac ischemic preconditioning. *Adv Drug Deliv Rev.* 2009 Nov 30;61(14):1324–31.

McKillop D, Pentieva K, Daly D, et al. The effect of different cooking methods on folate retention in various foods that are amongst the major contributors to folate intake in the UK diet. *Br J Nutr.* 2002;88(6):681–8.

Moraes FA, Cota AM, Campos FM, Pinheiro-Sant'Ana HM. Vitamin C loss in vegetables during storage, preparation and distribution in restaurants. *Cien Saude Colet.* 2010 Jan;15(1):51–62.

Nascimento OV, Boleti AP, Yuyama LK, Lima ES. Effects of diet supplementation with Camu-camu (Myrciaria dubia HBK McVaugh) fruit in a rat model of diet-induced obesity. *An Acad Bras Cienc.* 2013 March;85(1):355-63.

National Academy of Sciences, Institute of Medicine, Food and Nutrition Board. *Dietary Reference Intakes for Vitamin A, Vitamin K, Arsenic, Boron, Chromium, Copper, Iodine, Iron, Manganese, Molybdenum, Nickel, Silicon, Vanadium, and Zinc* (2001)

Okano T, Nakagawa K, Kamao M. In vivo metabolism of vitamin K: in relation to the conversion of vitamin $K_1$ to MK-4. *Clin Calcium.* 2009 Dec;19(12):1779–87.

Prakash, P., Russell, R. M., Krinsky, N. I. In vitro inhibition of proliferation of estrogen-dependent and estrogen-independent human breast cancer cells treated with carotenoids or retinoids. *The Journal of Nutrition*, 131(5), 1574–1580.

Rao AV, Agarwal S. Role of lycopene in cancer and heart disease. *Journal of the American College of Nutrition.* 2000;19(5):563–569.

Rock CL, Jacob RA, Bowen PE. Update on the biological characteristics of the antioxidant micronutrients: vitamin C, vitamin E, and the carotenoids. *J Am Diet Assoc.* 1996 Jul;96(7):693-702; quiz 703–4.

Said HM. Cell and molecular aspects of human intestinal biotin absorption. *J Nutr.* 2009 Jan;139(1):158–62.

Sato T, Schurgers LJ, Uenishi K. Comparison of menaquinone-4 and menaquinone-7 bioavailability in healthy women. *Nutr J.* 2012 Nov 12;11:93.

Schagen SK, Zampeli VA, Makrantonaki E, Zouboulis CC. Discovering the link between nutrition and skin aging. *Dermatoendocrinol.* 2012 Jul 1;4(3):298–307.

Shearer MJ, Newman P. Metabolism and cell biology of vitamin K. *Thromb Haemost.* 2008 Oct;100(4):530–47.

Shinmura K. Effects of caloric restriction on cardiac oxidative stress and mitochondrial bioenergetics: potential role of cardiac sirtuins. *Oxid Med Cell Longev.* 2013;2013:528935. doi: 10.1155/2013/528935. Epub 2013 Mar 18.

Sin HP, Liu DT, Lam DS. Lifestyle modification, nutritional and vitamins supplements for age-related macular degeneration. *Acta Ophthalmol.* 2013;91(1):6-11.

Stahl W, Heinrich U, Aust O, Tronnier H, Sies H. Lycopene-rich products and dietary photoprotection. *Photochem Photobio Sci.* 2006;5:238–242.

Suárez-Suárez A, Tovar-Sánchez A, Rosselló-Mora R. Determination of cobalamins (hydroxo-, cyano-, adenosyl- and methyl-cobalamins) in seawater using reversed-phase liquid chromatography with diode-array detection. *Anal Chim Acta.* 2011 Sep 2;701(1):81–5.

Tanumihardjo SA. Factors influencing the conversion of carotenoids to retinol: bioavailability to bioconversion to bioefficacy. *Int J Vitam Nutr Res.* 2002 Jan;72(1):40–5.

Thijssen HH, Vervoort LM, Schurgers LJ, Shearer MJ. Menadione is a metabolite of oral vitamin K. *Br J Nutr.* 2006 Feb;95(2):260–6.

Tucker KL, Rich S, Rosenberg I, et al. Plasma vitamin B-12 concentrations relate to intake source in the Framingham Offspring study. *Am J Clin Nutr.* 2000 Feb;71(2):514–22.

Vermeer C, Braam L. Role of K vitamins in the regulation of tissue calcification. *J Bone Miner Metab.* 2001;19(4):201–6.

Watanabe F. Vitamin $B_{12}$ sources and bioavailability. *Exp Biol Med* (Maywood). 2007;232(10): 1266–74.

Watanabe J, Oki T, Takebayashi J, et al. Improvement of the Lipophilic-Oxygen Radical Absorbance Capacity (L-ORAC) Method and Single-Laboratory Validation. *Biosci Biotechnol Biochem.* 2013 Apr 23;77(4):857–9.

Weaver CM, Heaney RP. *Calcium in Human Health.* Totowa, NJ. W.B. Humana Press, 2006.

Yang F, Tan HM, Wang H. Hyperhomocysteinemia and atherosclerosis. *Sheng Li Xue Bao.* 2005 Apr 25;57(2):103–14.

Zhong M, Kawaguchi R, Kassai M, Sun H. Retina, retinol, retinal and the natural history of vitamin A as a light sensor. *Nutrients.* 2012 Dec 19;4(12):2069–96.

**Choline**

National Nutrient Database for Standard Reference Release 27. ndb.nal.usda.gov/ndb/nutrients/index.

"Self Nutrition Data: Know What You Eat," Condé Nast, Inc. nutritiondata.self.com/facts/fats-and-oils/592/2.


**Chapter 7: Water and Hydration**

National Academy of Sciences. Institute of Medicine. Food and Nutrition Board. "Dietary Reference Intakes: Electrolytes and Water." fnic.nal.usda.gov/dietary-guidance/dietary-reference-intakes/dri-tables.

US Department of Agriculture, Center for Nutrition Policy and Promotion. "Sodium, Potassium, and Water." origin.www.cnpp.usda.gov/DGAs2010-DGACReport.htm.


**Chapter 8: The Effect of Heat on Nutrients and Enzymes**

**Heat and the Nutrient Content of Foods**

Bernhardt S, Schlich E. Impact of different cooking methods on food quality: Retention of lipophilic vitamins in fresh and frozen vegetables. *J Food Eng.* 2006;77(2):327–333.

Chai W, Liebman M. Effect of different cooking methods on vegetable oxalate content. *J Agric Food Chem.* 2005;53(8):3027–30.

Galgano F, Favati F, Caruso M, Pietrafesa A, Natella S. The influence of processing and preservation on the retention of health-promoting compounds in broccoli. *J Food Sci.* 2007;72(2):S130–5.

Gliszczynska-Swiglo A, Ciska E, Pawlak-Lemanska K, Chimielewski J, Borkowski T, Tyrakowska B. Changes in the content of health-promoting compounds and antioxidant activity of broccoli after domestic processing. *Food Addit Contam.* 2006;23(11):1088–98.

Hotz C, Gibson R. Traditional food processing and preparation practices to enhance the bioavailability of micronutrients in plant-based diets. *J Nutr.* 2007;137(4):1097–100.

Kimura M, Itokawa Y, Fujiwara M. Cooking losses of thiamin in food and its nutritional significance. *J Nutr Sci Vitaminol* (Tokyo);36 Suppl 1;S17–24.

Leskova E, Kubikova E, Kovacicova, Porubska J, Holcicova K. Vitamin Losses: Retention during heat treatment and continual changes expressed by mathematical models. *Journal of Food Composition and Analysis.* 2006;19(1):252–276.

Link L, Potter J. Raw versus cooked vegetables and cancer risk. *Cancer Epidemiol Biomarkers Prev.* 2004;13(9):1422–35.

Lopez-Berenguer C, Carvajal M, Moreno D, Garcia-Viguera C. Effects of microwave cooking conditions on bioactive compounds present in broccoli inflorescences. *J Agric Food Chem.* 2007;55(24):10001–7.

McKillop DJ, Pentieva K, Daly D, et al. The effect of different cooking methods on folate retention in various foods that are amongst the major contributors to folate intake in the UK diet. *Br J Nutr.* 2002;88(6):681–8.

Miglio C, Chiavaro E, Visconti A, Fogliano V, Pellegrini N. Effects of different cooking methods on nutritional and physiochemical characteristics of selected vegetables. *J Agric Food Chem.* 2008;56(1):139–47.

Paulus K. Changes in nutritional quality of food in catering. *J Nutr Sci Vitaminol* (Tokyo). 1990;36 Suppl 1:S35–44; discussion S44–5.

Petersen M. Influence of sous vide processing, steaming and boiling on vitamin retention and sensory quality in broccoli florets. *Z Lebensm Unters Forsch*. 1993;197(4):375–80.

Reddy M, Love M. The impact of food processing on the nutritional quality of vitamins and minerals. *Adv Exp Med Biol*. 1999;459:99–106.

Rumm-Kreuter D, Demmel I. Comparison of vitamin losses in vegetables due to various cooking methods. *J Nutr Sci Vitaminol* (Tokyo). 1990;Suppl 1;S7–14; discussion S14–5.

Steinhart H and Rathjen T. Dependence of tocopherol stability on different cooking procedures of food. *Int J Nutr Res* 2003;73(2):144–151.

Yuan G, Sun B, Yuan J, Wang Q. Effects of different cooking methods on health-promoting compounds of broccoli. *J Zhejiang Univ Sci B*. 2009;10(8):580–8.

## Enzymes

Barros M, Fleuri L, Macedo G. Seed lipases: sources, applications, and properties – a review. *Brazilian Journal of Chemical Engineering*. 2010;27(1):15-29.

Conaway CC, Getahun SM, Liebes LL, et al. Disposition of glucosinolates and sulforaphane in humans after ingestion of steamed and fresh broccoli. *Nutr Cancer*. 2000;38(2):168–78.

Cutler RR, Wilson P. Antibacterial activity of a new, stable, aqueous extract of allicin against methicillin-resistant Staphylococcus aureus. *Br J Biomed Sci*. 2004;61(2):71–4.

Getahun SM, Chung FL. Conversion of glucosinolates to isothiocyanates in humans after ingestion of cooked watercress. *Cancer Epidemiol Biomarkers Prev*. 1999 May;8(5):447–51.

Gliszczynska-Swiglo A, Ciska E, Pawlak-Lemanska K, Chimielewski J, Borkowski T, Tyrakowska B. Changes in the content of health-promoting compounds and antioxidant activity of broccoli after domestic processing. *Food Addit Contam*. 2006;23(11):1088–98.

Hirsch A, Forch K, Neidhart S, Wolf G, Carle R. Effects of thermal treatments and storage on pectin methylesterase and peroxidase activity in freshly squeezed orange juice. *J Agric Food Chem*. 2008;56(14):5691–9.

Howard LA, Jeffery EH, Wallig MA, Klein BP. Retention of phytochemicals in fresh and processed broccoli. *Journal of Food Science*. 1997;62(6):1098–1104.

Lee YM, Gweon OC, Seo YJ, et al. Antioxidant effect of garlic and aged black garlic in animal model of type 2 diabetes mellitus. *Nutr Res Pract*. 2009;3(2):156–61.

Link L, Potter J. Raw versus cooked vegetables and cancer risk. *Cancer Epidemiol Biomarkers Prev*. 2004;13(9):1422–35.

Modem S, Dicarlo SE, Reddy TR. Fresh Garlic Extract Induces Growth Arrest and Morphological Differentiation of MCF7 Breast Cancer Cells. *Genes Cancer*. 2012 Feb;3(2):177–86.

Mithen R, Dekker M, Verkerk R, Rabot S, Johnson I. The nutritional significance, biosynthesis and bioavailability of glucosinolates in human foods. *J Sci Food Agric*. 2000;80:967–84.

Navarro SL, Li F, Lampe JW. Mechanisms of action of isothiocyanates in cancer chemoprevention: an update. *Food Funct*. 2011 Oct;2(10):579–87.

Roxas M. The role of enzyme supplementation in digestive disorders. *Altern Med Rev*. 2008 Dec;13(4):307-14.

Shapiro TA, Fahey JW, Wade KL, Stephenson KK, Talalay P. Human metabolism and excretion of cancer chemoprotective glucosinolates and isothiocyanates of cruciferous vegetables. *Cancer Epidemiol Biomarkers Prev*. 1998 Dec;7(12):1091–100.

Song K, Milner J. The influence of heating on the anticancer properties of garlic. *J Nutr* 2001;131:1054–7S.

Stanley D, Farnden K, MacRae E. Plant α-amylases: functions and roles in carbohydrate metabolism. *Biologia*. 2005;60(Suppl. 16):65-71.

Tipton K, Boyce S. History of the enzyme nomenclature system. *Bioinformatics.* 2000 Jan;16(1):34–40.

Worthington Biochemical. *Manual of Clinical Enzyme Measurements.* Lakewood, NJ. 1972.

## Chapter 9: Understanding Calorie Density and Macronutrient Percentages

Atkinson F, Foster-Powell K, Brand-Miller J. International tables of glycemic index and glycemic load values: 2008. *Diabetes Care.* 2008;31(12):2281–3.

Ello-Martin J, Roe L, Ledikwe J, Beach A, Rolls B. Dietary energy density in the treatment of obesity: a year-long trial comparing 2 weight loss diets. *Am J Clin Nutr.* 2007;85(6):1465–77.

Ferrua MJ, Singh RP. Modeling the fluid dynamics in a human stomach to gain insight of food digestion. *J Food Sci.* 2010 Sep;75(7):R151–62.

Foster-Powell K, Holt S, Brand-Miller J. International table of glycemic index and glycemic load values: 2002. *Am J Clin Nutr.* 2002;76(1):5–56.

Johnson LR. *Essential Medical Physiology,* 2nd Edition. Philadelphia, PA: Lippincott-Raven Publishers, 1998.

Ledikwe J, Blanck H, Khan L, et al. Low-energy-density diets are associated with high diet quality in adults in the United States. *J Am Diet Assoc.* 2006;106(8):1172–80.

Ledikwe J, Ello-Martin J, Rolls B. Portion sizes and the obesity epidemic. *J Nutr.* 2005; 135(4):905–9.

Ledikwe J, Rolls B, Smiciklas-Wright H, et al. Reductions in dietary energy density are associated with weight loss in overweight and obese participants in the PREMIER trial. *Am J Clin Nutr.* 2007;85(5):1212–21.

Novotny JA, Gebauer SK, Baer DJ. Discrepancy between the Atwater factor predicted and empirically measured energy values of almonds in human diets. Am J Clin Nutr. 2012 Aug;96(2):296-301.

Rolls B, Barnett R. *Volumetrics: Feel Full on Fewer Calories.* New York, NY: Harper Collins Publishers, 2000.

———. *The Volumetrics Weight-Control Plan.* New York, NY: Harper Collins Publishers, 2000.

Zou ML, Moughan PJ, Awati A, Livesey G. Accuracy of the Atwater factors and related food energy conversion factors with low-fat, high-fiber diets when energy intake is reduced spontaneously. Am J Clin Nutr. 2007 Dec;86(6):1649-56.

## Chapter 10: Nutrient Analyses of Various Raw Food Diets

American Dietetic Association; Dietitians of Canada. Position of the American Dietetic Association and Dietitians of Canada: Vegetarian diets. *J Am Diet Assoc.* 2003 Jun;103(6):748-65.

Gallup, Inc. "In U.S., 5% Consider Themselves Vegetarians." conducted July 9–12, 2012. gallup.com/poll/156215/consider-themselves-vegetarians.aspx

## Chapter 11: The Importance of Focusing on Whole Plant Foods

John S, Sorokin AV, Thompson PD. Phytosterols and vascular disease. *Curr Opin Lipidol.* 2007 Feb;18(1):35–40.

Risérus U, Willett WC, Hu FB. Dietary fats and prevention of type 2 diabetes. *Prog Lipid Res.* 2009 Jan;48(1):44–51.

Simopoulos AP. The importance of the ratio of omega-6/omega-3 essential fatty acids. *Biomed Pharmacother.* 2002;56(8):365–79.

Storlien LH, Pan DA, Kriketos AD, et al. Skeletal muscle membrane lipids and insulin resistance. *Lipids.* 1996 Mar;31 Suppl:S261–5.

### Nutritional composition of chia seed oil

livingtreecommunity.com/store2/product.
asp?id=218,

therawfoodworld.com/running-man-raw-virgin-
chia-oil-12oz-running-food-pi1004193

## Chapter 12: Principles of Food Combining

### Food Combining Philosophy

Shelton HM. *The Science and Fine Art of Food and Nutrition*. Oldsmar, Florida: Natural Hygiene Press, 1984.

——. *Superior Nutrition*. San Antonio, Texas: Willow Publishing, 1987 (14th printing).

Wigmore A. *The Hippocrates Diet and Health Program*. Wayne, New Jersey: Avery Publishing Group Inc., 1984.

### Food Combining Research and Physiology

Guyton, AC. *Textbook of Medical Physiology*, 8th Edition. Philadelphia, PA: W.B. Saunders Company, 1991.

Groff JL and Gropper SS. *Advanced Nutrition and Human Metabolism*, 3rd Edition. Belmont, CA: Wadsworth Thomson Learning, 2000.

Weber E, Ehrlein HJ. Composition of enteral diets and meals providing optimal absorption rates of nutrients in mini pigs. *Am J Clin Nutr*. 1999;69(3):556–63.

## Chapter 13: Raw for Life: Helpful Raw-Food Success Strategies

Foster-Powell K, Holt S, Brand-Miller J. International table of glycemic index and glycemic load values: 2002. *Am J Clin Nutr*. 2002;76(1):5–56.

# Index

NOTE: Page references in *italics* refer to figures and tables.

## A

A, vitamin (retinol), 96–100, *97, 98, 99*
absorption
    of calcium, 72–73
    cooking and, 109
    digestion and, 169
    of iron, *77, 77*–78, 84
    of lycopene, 97, 100
    of vitamins, 87, 96
activity factor, *127,* 127–128
adenosylcobalamin, 88
adequate intakes (AIs)
    minerals, 71
    water, 105, *105*
adzuki beans, protein and amino acids in, *63*
agave syrup, dried agave compared to,
        156–157, *157–158*
algae, defined, 8
allicin, 115
alliinase, 115
almonds
    amino acid content of, *41*
    Basic Almond Loaf, 124, 125
alpha-linolenic acid (ALA), 22
amaranth
    protein and amino acids in, 56, *56, 58*
    as pseudograin, 7–8
*American Journal of Clinical Nutrition, 77,* 88

amino acids. *see also* protein; whole plant foods
    in fruits, 42, *42, 43, 44*
    in high-sweet fruit diet, *133*
    in intermediate raw diet sample menu, *140*
    in low-sweet fruit diet, 134, *137*
    in nuts and seeds, 39, *39, 40, 41*
    overview, 29
    in standard Western sample menu, *145*
    in vegetables, 33–34, *34, 35, 36, 37, 38*
amylase, 113, 170
anemia, 74. *see also* iron
animal products
    animal welfare and, 2, 177
    carbohydrates and, 9
    fat and, 25, 27, 28
    meat and calorie density, 122
    minerals and, 74, 85
    nutrient analyses of various diets, 130, 143
    omega-6 fats and, 25, *26*
    protein and, 29, 166
    raw, 3
    transitioning from Western diet to raw
        diet, 125, 147–148
    unsaturated fats and, 23, *24*
    vitamins and, 96, 102
*Annals of Nutrition and Metabolism,* 88
antioxidants. *see also* minerals; vitamins
    enzymes and, 114
    fat and, 21
arachidonic acid (AA), 22

# B

bananas, amino acid content of, *43*

barley, protein and amino acids in, *56, 57, 61*

basal metabolic rate (BMR), 127

*Basic Almond Loaf*

    calorie density of, 125

    recipe, 124

*Basic Green Smoothie*

    calorie density of, 125

    recipe, 124

beans, protein in, *62, 62–65, 63, 64, 65*

beta-carotene, 96

biotin (vitamin H, vitamin B$_7$), 92, *93*

blood, pH balance of, 84, *84*

blood sugar

    effect of carbohydrates on, 13–15

    glucose, defined, 9

blueberries, amino acid content in, *43*

body weight

    calories needed and, 126–127

    protein intake and, 30–32, *31*

bok choy, amino acid content in, *38*

boron, 72–73

Brazil nuts, 163

breads, water content of, *108*

*British Journal of Nutrition*, 110

broccoli

    amino acid content, *37*

    heating methods and, 110, 111, 114–115

brown rice

    protein and amino acids in, *56, 56, 57, 61*

    water content of, 108

buckwheat

    protein and amino acids in, *56, 56, 59*

    as pseudograin, 7–8

B vitamins

    B$_1$ (thiamin, thiamine), 89, *89*

    B$_2$ (riboflavin), 89–90, *90*

    B$_3$ (niacin), 90, *91*

    B$_5$ (pantothenic acid), 90–91, *91*

    B$_7$ (biotin, vitamin H), 92, *93*

    B$_6$ (pyridoxine), 91–92, *92*

    B$_9$ (folate, folic acid), 92–93, *93*, 110

    B$_{12}$ (cobalamin), 87–89

    choline, 94, *94*

# C

C, vitamin, *77*, 94–95, *95*

cabbage

    amino acid content in, *37*

    amino acid content in bok choy, *38*

    calcium in, 71

    enzymes in, 114

cacao butter, macronutrients in, *5, 6*

calcium

    absorption of, 72–73

    balance, 73, *73*

    content of, in various raw foods, *72*

    in high-sweet fruit diet, 130–131

    overview, 71

    sources of, 71

    vitamin D and, 100

calorie density, 117–128. *see also* calories

    applying, to foods and menus, 120–123

    calculating macronutrient percentage, 117–120

of common sweeteners, *121*

computing calorie needs, 126–128

computing calorie needs with activity factor, *127*, 127–128

examples, *123*, 123–125, *126*

importance of eating enough, 117, 125–126

overview, 117

of various foods and food groups, *120*

of various legumes/legume sprouts, *121*

calories

defined, 4

protein intake and, 32, *33*

types of raw food diet and, 3

in vegetables, 5

camu camu, 95

*Cancer Epidemiology, Biomarkers and Prevention*, 100

cantaloupes, amino acid content in, *44*

carbohydrates, 9–19. *see also* whole plant foods

calculating macronutrient percentage and, 117–118

defined, 4

digestion of, 113

disaccharides, *9*, 9–11

fiber and, 11–12, *12*

fructose compared to high-fructose corn syrup, 18–19

glycemic index, 13–15, *14*, *15*

glycemic load, *16*, 16–18, *18*

macronutrients, defined, 3–4

misconceptions about, 12

monosaccharides, 9–11, *10*

need for, 19

obesity and, 12

polysaccharides, 11

in processed foods, *13*

carotenoids, 96–100, *97*, *98*, *99*

carrots

amino acid content, *35*

glycemic index and, 15

cashews, amino acid content in, *41*

cauliflower, amino acid content in, *37*

celery, sodium in, 81, 82

Centers for Disease Control, 81

chia seeds

amino acid content, *40*

chia seed oil compared to, 154–155, *155–156*

chickpeas, protein and amino acids in, *63*

chlorophyll, 79–80

cholecalciferol, 100–101

choline, 94, *94*

cobalamin (vitamin $B_{12}$), 87–89

coconut oil

coconut meat compared to, 148–150, *149–150*

macronutrients in, 5, *6*

conversion factors, 178

cooking. *see also* heat

80-percent raw (20-percent cooked) diet, 3

heat and protein bioavailability, 68–69

methods used in raw diet, 2

raw *versus* cooked vegetables, 111–112

water content in cooked vegan foods, 107–108

copper, 84

corn

    amino acid content, *38*

    human milk compared to, *66–68, 67, 68*

cucumbers, as fruits, 5

cyanobacteria, 8

cyanocobalamin, 88

cysteine, 31

# D

D, vitamin, *72–73, 100,* 100–101

DASH (Dietary Approaches to Stopping
        Hypertension), 85–86

dietary fat. *see* fat

dietary fiber, defined, 4

Dietary Reference Intake (DRI)

    choline, 94

    copper, 84

    defined, 71

    essential fatty acids, 24

    iron, *74*

    macronutrients, 130

    manganese, 84

    resources, 179

    vitamin A (retinol), 97

    vitamin $B_1$ (thiamin), 89

    vitamin $B_2$ (niacin), 90

    vitamin $B_5$ (pantothenic acid), 91

    vitamin $B_6$ (pyridoxine), 92

    vitamin $B_7$ (biotin), 92

    vitamin $B_9$ (folate), 93

    vitamin $B_{12}$ (thiamin), 88

    vitamin C, 95

vitamin E, 102

vitamin K, 103

water, 108

digestion

    enzymes and, 112–115

    food combining and, *168–172, 171*

di-homo-gamma-linolenic acid (DGLA), 22

Dina, Karin, 2, *177*

Dina, Rick, 2, *177*

disaccharides, *9,* 9–11

docosahexaenoic acid (DHA), 22

double bonds, 21, 22

# E

E, vitamin, 101–102, *102,* 111

egg whites, effect of heat on, 68

eicosapentaenoic acid (EPA), 22

80-percent raw (20-percent cooked) diet

    defined, 3

    nutrient analysis of, *140,* 140–143, *142*

energy. *see also* calorie density

    as fat, 21

    obtaining sufficient calories, 117,
        125–126

enzymes

    enzymatic activity in food, 112–115

    food combining and enzyme cancellation
        concept, 170

essential fatty acids

    inflammation and, 23, 26–27

    maintaining omega-6 to omega-3 bal-
        ance, 23–25

    omega-3 fats, overview, 22–25

omega-6 fats, overview, 22–25

omega-9 fats, overview, 26–28

omega fat content in sample menus, compared, *146*

overview, 21–22

selected foods, high in omega-6 fats, *26*

selected foods, high in omega-9 fats, *27*

selected foods, with desirable ratio of omega-3 to omega-6 fats, *24*

standard Western diet compared to raw diets, 143

in typical salad and dressing, 25

*Experimental Biology and Medicine*, 88

## F

family/friends, support of, 174

fat, 21–28. *see also* whole plant foods

calculating macronutrient percentage and, 117–118

defined, 4

digestion of, 113

energy and, 21

essential fatty acids, overview, 21–22

food combining for, 166, 168

macronutrients, defined, 3–4

maintaining omega-6 to omega-3 balance, 23–25, *24, 26*

nutrient analyses of raw food diets, 143–144

omega-9, 26–28, *27*

saturated, sources, 27

saturated and unsaturated types, 21

fat-soluble vitamins

A (retinol), 96–100, *97, 98, 99*

D, 72–73, *100*, 100–101

E, 101–102, *102*, 111

heat and, 110

K, 13, *103*

overview, 96

fiber

calorie density and, 117, 121

defined, 11

glycemic index and, 17

as prebiotic, 11–12

fish. *see* animal products

flaxseeds

amino acid content, *40*

flax oil compared to, 152–153, *153–154*

flexibility, importance of, 173

folate (folic acid, vitamin $B_9$), 92–93, *93*, 110

Food and Drug Administration (FDA), 96

food combining, 165–172

basic principles of, 165–167

digestion and, 168–172, *171*

digestive pH and, 170–171, *171*

enzyme cancellation concept, 170

for fruits, 165–166, 167, 169

phases of food metabolism and, 168

for protein, starch, and fat, 166, 168

timing and, 172

for vegetables, 166, 168

food enzymes, 113–114

Framingham Offspring Study, 88

Framingham Osteoporosis Study, 86

free radicals, 21

fructooligosaccharides (FOS), 11–12, *12*

fructose

  defined, 9

  on glycemic index, 14

  high-fructose corn syrup compared to, 18–19, *19*

fruits. *see also individual names of fruits*

  amino acids in, 42, *42, 43, 44*

  calorie density of, 120

  defined, 5

  food combining for, 165–166, 167, 169

  glycemic value of, *14*

  nutrient comparison of whole plant foods, *158–159, 158–162, 160–161*

frying, of foods, 110

## G

galactose, 9

*Garden Vegetable Salad*

  calorie density of, 123–124

  nutrients in, compared to *Raw Chocolate Pie*, 162, *162–163*

  recipe, 123

  vitamins and minerals in, *126*

garlic, enzymes and, 115

"Generally Recognized as Safe," 96

glucose

  defined, 9

  on glycemic index, 14

  high-fructose corn syrup and, 18–19

glucosinolates, 114–115

glycemic index (GI)

  creation of, 13

digestion and, 168–169

glycemic load, defined, 16

glycemic load of selected whole foods and process foods, *18*

glycemic load *versus, 16,* 16–18

  of selected fruits, *14*

  of selected whole foods and processed foods, *15*

grains

  calorie density and, 121–122

  defined, 7–8

  grass botanical family, 7, 8, 54, *54, 55*

  protein in, 55–62, *56, 57, 58, 59, 60, 61*

  pseudograins, defined, 7–8

  wheat, *58, 60,* 66–68, *67, 68*

grass. *see also* grains

  botanical family of, defined, 7, 8

  spirulina, 54, *54, 55*

Greenberg, James, 23

green peas, protein and amino acids in, *64*

*Green Smoothie. see also Basic Green Smoothie*

  nutrients in, compared to *Raw Chocolate Pie*, 159–162, *160–161*

  recipe, 161

## H

Harris-Benedict equation, 126–127

Harvard Health Publications, 81

heat

  enzymatic activity in food and, 112–115

  minerals and, 109

protein availability and, 68–69

raw *versus* cooked vegetables, 111–112

vitamins and, 109–111

HFCS 55, 18–19, *19*

high-fructose corn syrup, 18–19, *19*

high-sweet fruit diet

defined, 3

nutrient analysis of, 130–133, *131, 132, 133*

protein and amino acids in, 44–45, *46, 47*

water and, 105–106

Holick, Michael, 101

Howell, Edward, 113

human milk, corn and wheat compared to, 66–68, *67, 68*

hydroxocobalamin, 88

# I

iceberg lettuce, amino acid content in, *36*

inflammation

omega-3 and omega-6 fats, 23

omega-9 fats and, 26–27

Institute of Medicine (IOM), 71, 80, 81, 105

insulin

carbohydrates and, 13

glucose and, 13

intermediate raw diet (moderate fruit-moderate fat)

defined, 3

nutrient analysis of, 137–138, *139, 140*

protein and amino acids in, 51–54, *52, 53*

water and, 106

*International Journal for Vitamin and Nutrition Research*, 88

inulin, 11–12, *12*

iron

absorption, *77, 77*–78, 84

balance, 75–76, *76*

content of, in selected raw foods, *75*

forms of, 74

overview, 74

sources of, 74

isothiocyanates, 114

# J

Jenkins, David, 13

*Journal of Nutrition*, 85, 115

# K

K, vitamin, 13, *103*

kale, amino acid content in, *37*

Kamut, protein and amino acids in, *59*

kelp

amino acid content, *55*

defined, 8

kidney beans, protein and amino acids in, *64*

Kobe Pharmaceutical University (Japan), 103

# L

labels, reading, 118

lactase, 112

lactose, 9, 112

legumes

calorie density and, 121

defined, 8

legumes/legume sprouts and calorie density, *121*

protein and amino acids in lentils, *64*

lentils, protein and amino acids in, *64*

lettuce, amino acid content in, *36*

lima beans, protein and amino acids in, *63*

linoleic acid (LA), 22

lipase, 113, 170

long-chain saturated fats (LCSFs), 27

low-sweet fruit diet

    defined, 3

    nutrient analysis of, 133–136, *136, 137*

    protein and amino acids in, 47–48, *49,*
        *50*

    water and, 106

lutein, 97–98, *99*

lycopene, 98–100, *99*

lysine. *see also* amino acids

    effect of heat on, 68–69

    overview, 56

# M

macadamia nuts, amino acid content in, 39,
    *40*

macronutrients. *see also* carbohydrates; fat;
    fiber; protein

    calorie density and calculating macronutri-
        ent percentage, 117–121

    defined, 3–4

    in 80-percent raw menu (20-percent
        cooked), sample menu, *140*

    in high-sweet fruit diet, *133*

    in high-sweet fruit diet, sample menu, *131*

    in intermediate raw diet, sample menu,
        *139*

    in low-sweet fruit diet, sample menu, *136*

nutrient analyses of raw food diets and,
    130

    in whole plant foods, 4–8, *6–7*

magnesium

    in cholorphyll, 79–80

    content of, in various raw foods, *78*

    overview, 79

maltose, 9

manganese, 84

mango, amino acid content in, *43*

*Manual of Clinical Enzyme Measurements,*
    *The,* 112

measurement, conversion of, 178

meat. *see* animal products

medium-chain saturated fats (MCSFs), 27

Mendel, Lafayette, 66

metabolic enzymes, 113–114

metabolism, food combining and, 168

methionine, 31

methylcobalamin, 88

milk (human), corn and wheat compared to,
    66–68, *67, 68*

millet, protein and amino acids in, 56, *56, 57*

minerals, 71–86. *see also* whole plant foods

    calcium, 71–73, *72, 73*

    calorie density and, *126*

    copper, 84

    effect of heat on, 109

    in 80-percent raw menu (20-percent
        cooked) sample menu, *142*

    in high-sweet fruit diet sample menu, *132*

    in intermediate raw diet sample menu, *139*

    iron, 74–78, *75, 77*

in low-sweet fruit diet sample menu, *136*

magnesium, *78, 79*

magnesium and chlorophyll, 79–80

manganese, 84

pH balance and raw diet, *84,* 84–86

phytate content of various plant foods
    and, 76

potassium, 80

recommended intakes, 71

selenium, 82–83, *83*

sodium, 80–83, *82*

in standard Western sample menu, *145*

zinc, *83,* 83–84

monosaccharides, 9–11, *10*

monounsaturated fats, 21

Mozaffarian, Dariush, 24

myrosinase, 114

# N

napa cabbage, amino acid content in, *37*

National Academy of Sciences, 81

navy beans, protein and amino acids in, *65*

niacin (vitamin B$_3$), 90, *91*

nightshade family, as fruits, 5

nonstarchy vegetables, 5

nori, 8

Nurses' Health Study, 28

nutrient analyses of raw food diets, 129–146
    80-percent raw menu (20-percent
        cooked), *140,* 140–143, *142*
    essential fats in various menus, 143–144
    high-sweet fruit menu, 130–133, *131,*
        *132, 133*
    intermediate raw menu, 137–138, *139,*
        *140*

low-sweet fruit menu, 133–136, *136, 137*

macronutrient requirements, 130

overview, 129

resources, 179

standard Western menu, 143–146, *144,*
    *145*

nutrient analyses of whole plant foods
    chia seeds compared to chia seed oil,
        154–155, *155–156*
    coconut oil compared to coconut meat,
        148–150, *149–150*
    flaxseeds and flax oil, 152–153,
        *153–154*
    olive oil compared to olives, 148, 150,
        *151–152*

*Nutrition and Cancer,* 114

nuts
    amino acids in, 39, *39, 40, 41*
    *Basic Almond Loaf,* 124, *125*
    Brazil nuts as source of selenium, 163
    calorie density of, 121
    defined, 5

# O

oats, protein and amino acids in, *59*

obesity, carbohydrates and, 12, *13*

Ohio State University, 79

oils. *see also* fat
    chia seed oil compared to chia seeds,
        154–155, *155–156*
    coconut oil, macronutrients in, 5, *6*
    coconut oil compared to coconut meat,
        148–150, *149–150*
    defined, 5

flax oil compared to flaxseeds, 152–153, 153–154

olive oil, macronutrients in, 5, 6

olive oil compared to olives, 148, 150, 151–152

oligosaccharides, 11–12

olive oil

  macronutrients in, 5, 6

  olives compared to, 148, 150, 151–152

omega-3 and omega-6 fats

  inflammation and, 23

  maintaining balance of, 23–25, 24, 26

  overview, 22–25

  standard Western diet compared to raw diets, 143

omega-9 fats, 26–28, 27

oranges, amino acid content in, 43

Osborne, Thomas, 66

oxalic acid

  calcium and, 73, 73

  heat and, 109

  iron and, 77

**P**

palmitic acid, 27

pantothenic acid (vitamin B5), 90–91, 91

pH balance

  food combining and digestive pH, 170–171, 171

  minerals and, 84–86, 85

phenylalanine, 31

phytic acid (phytate)

  calcium and, 73

  heat and, 109

iron and, 77

overview, 75, 76

phytochemical activation, 114–115

pinto beans, protein and amino acids in, 64

Poaceae, 7

polysaccharides, 11

polyunsaturated fats, 21

potassium

  content of, in various foods, 81

  overview, 80

  sources of, 80

potato, amino acid content in, 35

powdered dried grass, 8

Poznan University (Poland), 110

prebiotic, fiber as, 11–12

processed foods

  minimizing or eliminating, 147–148

  overview, 1

  protein deficiency and, 65

product-based information, understanding, 175

proteases, 113–114, 170

protein, 29–69

  amino acids, in comparative menus, 133, 134, 137, 140, 145

  amino acids, in fruits, 42, 42, 43, 44

  amino acids, in nuts and seeds, 39, 39, 40, 41

  amino acids, in vegetables, 33–34, 34, 35, 36, 37, 38

  amino acids, overview, 29

  in beans, 62, 62–65, 63, 64, 65

  calculating macronutrient percentage and, 117–118

deficiency, 65–69, *67*

defined, 4

food combining for, 166, 168

in grains, 55–62, *56, 57, 58, 59, 60, 61*

in low-sweet fruit diet, 134

macronutrients, defined, 3–4

recommended intakes, 30–33, *31, 33*

in sample raw food diets, 44–54, *46, 47,*
*49, 50, 52, 53*

in sea vegetables and spirulina, 54, *54,*
*55*

"Protein and Amino Acid Requirements in Human Nutrition" (WHO), 30–31

pseudograins, defined, 7–8

pumpkin seeds

amino acid content, *41*

magnesium and, 79

Purdue University, 79

pyridoxine (vitamin B$_6$), 91–92, *92*

## Q

quinoa

protein and amino acids in, 56, *56, 58*

as pseudograin, 7–8

## R

*Raw Chocolate Pie*

nutrients in, compared to *Garden Veg-*
*etable Salad*, 162, *162–163*

nutrients in, compared to *Green Smoothie,*
159–162, *160–161*

recipe, 161

raw diet, 1–8. *see also* calorie density; carbohydrates; fat; heat; minerals; nutrient

analyses of raw food diets; protein;
success strategies; vitamins; whole
plant foods

benefits of, 1–2

defined, 2–3

importance of eating enough, 117,
125–126

macronutrients, overview, 3–8, *6–7*

understanding information about,
174–176

*Raw Salad and Dressing*, 25

recipes

*Basic Almond Loaf*, 124

*Basic Green Smoothie*, 124

*Garden Vegetable Salad*, 123

*Green Smoothie*, 161

*Raw Chocolate Pie*, 161

*Salad*, 25

*Salad Dressings*, 25, 123

Recommended Dietary Allowances (RDAs)

defined, 4

minerals, 71, 74, 82–83, 84

protein, 130

vitamins, 101

recommended intakes. *see also* minerals;
protein

minerals, 71

protein, 30–33, *31, 33*

Research Institute of Child Nutrition, 85

resources, 179

retinol activity equivalent (RAE), 96, *97*

retinol (vitamin A), 96–100, *97, 98, 99*

riboflavin (vitamin B$_2$), 89–90, *90*

rice

    protein and amino acids in, *56, 56,*
        *57, 61*

    water content of, 108

Rolls, Barbara, 120

romaine lettuce, amino acid content in, *36*

Rose, William, 66

Royal Veterinary and Agricultural University
        (Denmark), 110

rye, protein and amino acids in, *56, 57*

# S

*Salad Dressing. see also Garden Vegetable*
        *Salad*

    calorie density of, 123–124

    recipe, 123

    vitamins and minerals in, *126*

salad recipes, 25, 45, 123–124, *126*

sample menus

    80-percent raw menu (20-percent
        cooked), 141

    high-sweet fruit diet, 131

    intermediate raw diet, 138

    low-sweet fruit diet, 135

    standard Western, 144

saturated fats

    defined, 21

    sources of, 27

Schwalfenberg, Gerry, 23

Science of Raw Food Nutrition classes (Dina,
        Dina), 2, 177

sea vegetables, protein in, *54, 54, 55*

seeds

    amino acids in, *39, 39, 40, 41*

    calorie density of, 121

defined, 5

magnesium in pumpkin seeds, 79

oils of, 152–153, *153–154,* 154–155,
        *155–156*

selenium

    Brazil nuts as source of, 163

    content of, in various raw foods, 83

    overview, 82–83

Shelton, Herbert, 165

short-chain saturated fats (SCSFs), 27

Simopoulos, Artemis, 23

*Smoothie, Green,* 159–162, *160–161*

soaking

    iron absorption and, 77

    water content in foods and, 106

sodium

    content of, in various raw foods, *82*

    in low-sweet fruit diet, 134

    overview, 80–81

    potassium and, 80

soybeans, protein and amino acids in, *65*

spelt, protein and amino acids in, *59*

spinach

    amino acid content, *38*

    heating methods and, 110

spirulina

    amino acid content, *55*

    overview, 8

    protein in, *54, 54, 55*

sprouts

    defined, 8

    iron absorption and, 77

squash

    amino acid content, *35*

    as fruits, 5

standard Western menu

nutrient analysis of, 143–146, *144, 145*

transitioning to raw diet from, 125, 147–148 (*see also* whole plant foods)

starch

defined, 11

food combining for, 166, 168

starchy vegetables, 5

State University of Campinas (Brazil), 95

State University of Maring (Brazil), 95

steaming, of foods, 110

strawberries, amino acid content in, *44*

success strategies, 173–176

flexibility, 173

sharing diet with friends and family, 174

understanding information about raw food, 174–176

sucrose

on glycemic index, 14

high-fructose corn syrup and, 19

overview, 9, 10, *10*

sunflower plant family

calcium in, 71

sunflower seeds, amino acid content, *41*

sunlight, vitamin D and, *100,* 100–101

superfoods

beliefs about, 158

camu camu, 95

in 80-percent raw diet (20-percent cooked), 143

nutrient analyses for, 143

sweeteners

calorie density of, *121,* 123

nutrient comparison of whole plant foods, 156–157, *157–158*

sweet potato, amino acid content in, *35*

**T**

teff, protein and amino acids in, *58*

testing, for vitamin deficiencies, 88–89

thiamin (thiamine, vitamin $B_1$), 89, *89*

thyroid, selenium and, 82

Tohoku University (Japan), 103

tomato, amino acid content in, *36*

tyrosine, 31

**U**

University of Illinois, 66

University of Kyoto (Japan), 109

University of Maastricht (Netherlands), 103

University of North Carolina, 79

University of Parma (Italy), 110

University of Sydney (Australia), 13

unsaturated fats, 21

U.S. Department of Agriculture (USDA), 81, 118

U.S. Department of Health and Human Services (HHS), 81

**V**

vegan diet

vitamin A for, 96

vitamin $B_{12}$ for, 87–88

water content in cooked foods, 107–108

whole plant foods in, 157

vegetables. *see also individual names of vegetables*

amino acids in, 33–34, *34, 35, 36, 37, 38*

calorie density of, 120, 133

defined, 5

food combining for, 166, 168

*Garden Vegetable Salad,* 123–124, *126, 162, 162–163*

very long-chain saturated fats (VLCSFs), 27

vitamers, 102

*Vitamin D Solution, The* (Holick), 101

vitamins, 87–103. *see also* whole plant foods

A (retinol), 96–100, *97, 98, 99*

B₁ (thiamin, thiamine), 89, *89*

B₂ (riboflavin), 89–90, *90*

B₃ (niacin), 90, *91*

B₅ (pantothenic acid), 90–91, *91*

B₆ (pyridoxine), 91–92, *92*

B₇ (biotin, vitamin H), 92, *93*

B₉ (folate, folic acid), 92–93, *93*, 110

B₁₂ (cobalamin), 87–89

C, *77*, 94–95, *95*

calorie density and, *126*

choline, 94, *94*

D, 72–73, *100,* 100–101

E, 101–102, *102,* 111

effect of heat on, 109–111

in 80-percent raw menu (20-percent cooked) sample menu, *142*

fat-soluble, overview, 96

in high-sweet fruit diet sample menu, *132*

in intermediate raw diet sample menu, *139*

K, 13, *103*

in low-sweet fruit diet sample menu, *136*

in standard Western sample menu, *145*

testing for vitamin deficiencies, 88–89

water-soluble, overview, 87

## W

wakame, amino acid content in, *55*

water

calorie density and, 121

for hydration, *105,* 105–108, *107, 108*

water-soluble vitamins

B₁ (thiamin, thiamine), 89, *89*

B₂ (riboflavin), 89–90, *90*

B₃ (niacin), 90, *91*

B₅ (pantothenic acid), 90–91, *91*

B₆ (pyridoxine), 91–92, *92*

B₇ (biotin, vitamin H), 92, *93*

B₉ (folate, folic acid), 92–93, *93,* 110

B₁₂ (cobalamin), 87–89

C, *77*, 94–95, *95*

choline, 94, *94*

heat and, 110

overview, 87

wheat

human milk compared to, 66–68, *67, 68*

protein and amino acids in, *58*

wheat flour (refined, whole), protein and amino acids, *60*

white rice, protein and amino acids in, *61*

whole plant foods, 147–164

eating more whole foods for success, 157–164, *158–159, 160–161, 162–163*

importance of focusing on, 147–148

macronutrients in, 4–8, 6–7 (*see also*
carbohydrates; fat; protein)

nutrient comparisons of, 148–155, *149–*
*150, 151–152, 153–154,*
*155–156*

raw food sweeteners, 156–157,
*157–158*

Wigmore, Ann, 165

World Health Organization (WHO), 30–31.
*see also* nutrient analyses of raw
food diets; protein

## Z

zeaxanthin, 97–98, *99*

zinc

content of, in various raw foods, *83*

overview, 83–84

zucchini, amino acid content in, *36*

**Would you like to learn more about raw food nutrition?** Access these and many other learning opportunities through our website: **rawfoodeducation.com**

# RAW FOOD EDUCATION

**Science of Raw Food Nutrition—** a comprehensive, 100-hour curriculum, taught in person at Living Light International, the world's premiere raw vegan school, in Ft. Bragg, California. We make complex scientific concepts easy for the nonscientific person to understand and provide depth for  those who already have a science or nutrition background. Two levels of certification are offered.

 **Dr. Karin on Instagram:** Check out Dr. Karin's experiences with raw food, gardening, and related topics.

**Science of Raw Food Nutrition I Online Course:** The first twelve hours of our Science of Raw Food Nutrition curriculum is available as an online video course. This is a great way to  learn more in the comfort of your own home and experience the quality of our classes.

**Science of Raw Food Nutrition on Facebook:** Find links to articles written by Dr. Karin and Dr. Rick, some of their personal experience as long-term raw-  food enthusiasts, updates about raw food nutrition topics, links to videos, and more.

 **YouTube channels:** See and hear Dr. Karin and Dr. Rick present various science-related, raw food nutrition topics, as well as personal experiences as long-term raw-food enthusiasts.

 **Email newsletter:** Keep up to date with news on raw food nutrition topics, announcements about our classes and speaking engagements, and more.

 **Lab Testing and Consulting:** See if you're on the right track and discover which tests are most appropriate for you. **rawfoodconsulting.com**

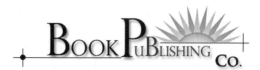

# BOOK PUBLISHING CO.

*books that educate, inspire, and empower*

To find your favorite books on plant-based cooking and nutrition,
living foods lifestyle, and healthy living, visit:
BookPubCo.com

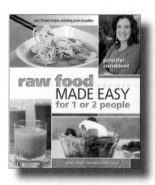

Raw Food Made Easy,
Revised Edition
*Jennifer Cornbleet*
978-1-57067-273-6 • $19.95

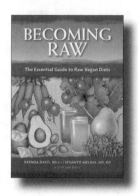

Becoming Raw
*Brenda Davis, RD,
Vesanto Melina, MS, RD,
Rynn Berry*
978-1-57067-305-4 • $16.95

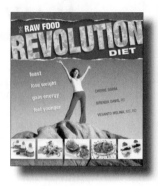

The Raw Food Revolution Diet
*Cherie Soria,
Brenda Davis, RD,
Vesanto Melina, Ms, RD*
978-1-57067-185-2 • $21.95

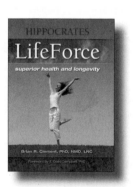

Hippocrates LifeForce
*Brian R. Clement, PhD, NMD, LNC*
978-1-57067-249-1 • $14.95

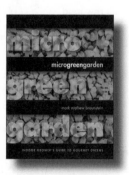

Microgreen Garden
*Mark Braunstein*
978-1-57067-294-1 • $14.95

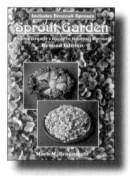

Sprout Garden,
Revised Edition
*Mark Braunstein*
978-1-57067-073-2 • $12.95

Purchase these health titles and cookbooks from your local bookstore or natural food store,
or you can buy them directly from:

Book Publishing Company • PO Box 99 • Summertown, TN 38483 • 1-888-260-8458

*Please include $3.95 per book for shipping and handling.*